Depression Anonymous
The Big Book on Depression Addiction

Dennis Ortman

For information, contact:

MSI Press
1760-F Airline Highway, 203
Hollister, CA 95023
Orders@MSIPress.com
Telephone/Fax: 831-886-2486

Library of Congress Control Number 2016935312

ISBN 9781942891260

cover design by Carl Leaver
cover photos: Shutterstock.com

Contents

Introduction...v

PART ONE
DEPRESSION AS AN ADDICTION 1

1. **The Many Faces of Depression**
    Living With Loss...3

2. **Depression as a Mood Addiction**
    Trying to Control the Uncontrollable.....................................13

3. **The Process of Addiction**
    Contending with Waves Of Loss..23

4. **The Addictive Personality**
    The Walking Dead...31

PART TWO
HOMECOMING...41

5. **The Steps**
    A Journey Home...43

6. **Defeated by Sorrow**
    Embracing the Pain 51

7. **Abundance**
    Coming to Faith...61

8. **Choose Life**
    Taking a Leap 73

9. **Night Vision**
    An Honest Look...83

10. **Lighten the Burden**
    Truth Telling 93

11. **Prepare the Way**
   A Humble Request 103

12. **Feeling Remorse**
   Forgiveness from the Heart..117

13. **Out of the Shadows**
   Seeing Clearly...131

14. **Grateful Abundance**
   Living Fully Now...143

15. **Share Life**
   Joyful Giving 155

   Epilogue
   The Journey Is Home...167

   Endnotes...173

   Suggested Readings 177

Introduction

> "Progress is impossible without change, and those who cannot change their minds cannot change anything."
>
> —George Bernard Shaw

Nothing remains the same. One constant in life is change. Some changes we initiate and welcome, but many come unannounced. Changes in health, finances, relationships, and even the weather occur, requiring stressful adjustments. In our driven society, the pace of change accelerates at a mind-numbing speed.

All change involves inevitable loss and anticipated gain. How do we react to these losses and gains? We naturally enjoy the gains, but may struggle with the losses. We grieve the loss of a comforting familiarity. We feel sadness. However, if we become stuck in our sorrow, become preoccupied with what could have been, without hope for a new life, we become depressed. Life loses its joy. The hope for happiness is dashed. Our depressed mood may progress to the point that we say to ourselves: "I'm powerless over my depression; my life has become unmanageable because of it." At the brink of despair, feeling possessed and powerless, our depression has become an addiction. It has become like a drug that takes over our lives.

LAURA'S STORY

"All I want to do is sleep," Laura, a woman in her sixties, lamented.

Her husband and son begged her to get out of bed and do something, do anything. "I don't have any interest in doing anything. Nothing gives me any pleasure anymore," she protested.

"You used to love to cook and sew," they reminded her. "Why don't you just try it?" Laura simply turned away and buried her head in the pillow.

Laura became depressed three years ago after suffering two blows. She was stunned when her doctor told her after a routine exam and subsequent biopsy that she had breast cancer. She told her husband and son the devastating news, but made them promise not to tell anyone else. Even though she considered her elderly mother her best friend, she did not want to tell her, reasoning to herself, "I don't want to worry her. She's so fragile and old."

Laura began chemotherapy for cancer and lost weight, and her hair. Somehow she deluded herself that she could hide the truth from her mother indefinitely. Then the second blow struck. Her eighty-five year old mother suddenly died of a heart attack. Laura's grief knew no bounds. After the initial shock that carried her through her mother's funeral, a dark cloud of depression enveloped her. Her already diminished appetite disappeared completely. She felt so exhausted that she only wanted to sleep. Family members visited, learning that she had cancer in addition to her grief, but she did not want to see anyone. She could only say, "I want to die and be with my mother."

Her supportive Polish family felt helpless to get her out of the mood that gripped her. They forced her to get out of bed and eat. They took her, against her will, to family gatherings where she sat in silence in a stuffed chair in the corner of the room, repelling any conversation. They took her to a psychiatrist for medication and to a psychologist for counseling. She reluctantly took the Effexor, Abilify, Xanax, and Provigil as the doctor prescribed. She listened passively to the advice of the doctors and her family and simply refused to do anything for herself. Her family, compassionate and frustrated, prodded her and waited on her. She continued to sleepwalk through her life.

Three years after the cancer diagnosis and her mother's death, the doctors told her that her cancer was in complete remission. Instead of feeling relief, Laura commented, "I don't believe it. I don't believe the cancer will ever leave me." She complained that she feared losing her mind because she could not escape her preoccupation with cancer. "It's eating me up inside," she said. She also refused to visit her mother's grave, explaining, "It would be just too painful."

It was not cancer that was consuming her. It was her depression and fear that were eating her alive.

DEPRESSION AS A DRUG

All of us feel blue from time to time. After all, sadness, sorrow, and grief are natural reactions to the loss of persons and things that are important to us. Feeling sad, we withdraw into a cocoon to soothe ourselves and adjust to the change in our life. We withdraw to nurse the wound of the loss. Feeling the pain, we inwardly search for its meaning, looking for a way of making sense of it. In this grieving process, we slowly let go of all the energy we used to put into what was lost and come to accept the void in our lives. If we do not succumb to the temptation of bitterness, the accepted pain of sorrow opens our hearts to new life and to empathy for others.

But sometimes the loss can seem unbearable and the sorrow overwhelming. The sadness reaches to the core of our being and a black cloud envelops us. We cannot escape the darkness. Our bodies, minds, and spirits become possessed. We cannot sleep or eat normally, and our energy dissipates. Joy flees our lives, and nothing gives us pleasure anymore. We begin to dread our daily routines and hate our lives. Despair grips us. We lose all hope for the future, entertaining thoughts of dying as an escape from the intolerable pain.

When we become stuck in sorrow and the black mood interferes with our happiness and daily living, we suffer from clinical depression.

If your depressed mood has interfered with your wellbeing for an extended period of time, you are not alone. Depression runs rampant in our fast-paced society. Nearly a fifth (19.3%) of adults and 14.3% of teens will suffer from clinical depression at some time during their lives (1). Women are twice as likely as men to experience a mood disorder. Depression is on the rise. Ten times more people have been diagnosed with it than two decades ago. What is most troubling about a mood disorder is its persistence. If you have had one depressive episode, the likelihood of you having another is 50%. After three episodes of depression, the lifetime risk of relapse is a staggering 90% (2).

If you suffer from depression, a persistent deep sadness, you may feel powerless to overcome it. Perhaps you have tried a variety of treatments: medication, counseling, self-help, or even electroshock therapy. You may have felt some relief, but the mood still seems to enslave you. If so, you may be addicted to your depressed mood. Here are some questions to ask yourself to determine if your mood is addictive:

- Do you feel overwhelmed often by a sense of loss and helplessness?
- Do you consider your sadness excessive, even crippling most of the time?
- Even though your depressed reactions are painful and harmful, do you feel powerless to stop them?
- Does your preoccupation with past hurts and regrets interfere with your life?
- Do you disengage from life, and feel like you are sleepwalking through it?
- Does your need to isolate seem excessive, interfering with your relationships?
- Do you feel hopeless about finding a cure for your depression?

Without realizing it, your depression acts like a drug that sedates, numbs, and possesses you.

You probably do not think of your depressed mood as a drug because it drains you of pleasure in life. You cannot imagine deriving any benefit from it. Nevertheless, depression acts like a sedative-hypnotic that lulls you to sleep. Under its influence, your body, mind, and spirit shut down. You lack energy and motivation to become engaged in life. You cannot eat or sleep as you did before. The arousal center in your brain is anesthetized so you cannot concentrate, remember, think clearly, or make decisions quickly. Your mind obsesses about regrets, disappointments, and your own worthlessness. You feel compelled to isolate yourself in your misery.

Most tragically, depression deadens your spirit. You no longer feel alive. You feel possessed by a "noonday demon" that wrings your soul of all hope, meaning, and the will to live. You are powerless in the grasp of this demon that rules your life.

The greatest loss in being depressed is the loss of yourself. You do not own your life. Your addictive illness does. Yet you are not beyond hope. Through recovery, you can come home to yourself.

HOMECOMING

Since depression afflicts the body, mind, and spirit, treatment must address the whole person. Most treatments, such as medication, cognitive-behavioral therapy, and self-help books encourage care of the body and mind. What is lacking is attention to the spirit, which languishes under the weight of depression. What can fill the gap?

Bill Wilson, the cofounder of Alcoholics Anonymous, suffered from both severe alcoholism and depression. Even after years of counseling, taking medications, and being hospitalized, he was still hopelessly depressed, suicidal, and drinking excessively. Bill met with a schoolboy friend who had become sober and turned his life around. Intrigued, Bill asked him his secret. His friend responded, "I got religion." Bill was shocked at what he heard. He was not a religious, church-going man. In fact, because he prided himself on his reasonableness, he had an aversion to religion and those who lived by a blind faith.

His friend explained that he had a spiritual conversion, a profound experience of God's presence in his life that transformed him internally. How you understand God is irrelevant, he said. What made a difference was the personal experience of something greater than himself. Bill experienced many believers as in-your-face, holier-than-thou, having-all-the-answers kinds of people. He was a searcher of truth who looked for answers that made sense to him. While listening to the quiet stirrings of his heart one day, Bill suddenly experienced a spiritual presence, a Power greater than himself that he had never noticed before. He felt transformed and did not crave drinking anymore. He then became convinced that a spiritual awakening was necessary to be freed from the bonds of addiction. Having achieved sobriety, he initiated the fellowship of Alcoholics Anonymous using the guidance of the Twelve Steps.

The Twelve Steps can offer you a path to awakening your spirit, which has been deadened by your depressed mood. The word depressed means "pressed down." What is pressed down is your life-giving spirit, which is the core of who you are. Your spirit, your soul, is connected to a Power greater than the self you recognize with your ordinary mind. Your spirit is connected with the whole universe, from which it draws its energy. The Steps provide guidance for your personal journey into the darkness of your depression so that you can discover your true self and release the Power within you. They are a way to come home to your authentic self.

Those who achieve a quality sobriety through the Steps insist on the essential importance of a spiritual conversion. Like Bill Wilson, you may balk at this requirement for healing and growth. Nearly twenty percent of Americans consider themselves atheists or agnostics, like Bill Wilson. Only about twenty percent attend religious services weekly (3). Perhaps you have been scandalized by the hypocrisy of church leaders, the clergy sex abuse scandal, and the mean-spiritedness of the abortion and gay and women's rights debates. Perhaps you have observed the narrow-mindedness, blind obedience, and immaturity of many professed believers. Religious practice seems to lead to personal transformation so rarely. Perhaps God talk irritates you in reducing the mystery of life to a handful of dogmas.

The Steps invite you to undertake a journey to recover your true spirit and to appreciate the sacred Light that shines through your dark moods. The Steps draw from ancient wisdom sources, offering practical guidance on living a good life, in clear, contemporary, straightforward language. This book is an adaptation of the Twelve Steps for finding freedom from your addiction to your depressed mood.

MY PERSONAL JOURNEY

My life can be almost neatly divided into two halves. I was raised Roman Catholic, entered the seminary at age fourteen, and was ordained a priest thirteen years later. I served in various parishes in the Archdiocese of Detroit for fourteen years. During that time, many parishioners came to me in times of crisis. I counseled them the best I could and referred them to professionals. I heard their confessions and offered God's forgiveness. In my experience, many of those I served were preoccupied with sin and guilt and sought forgiveness and a life of greater holiness.

At age forty, at midlife, I left the active ministry to be married. In making that decision, I prayed, sought counseling, and searched my soul for divine guidance. For a second career, I entered the clinical psychology program at the University of Detroit-Mercy and obtained a doctoral degree. Ironically, the psychology program at that Jesuit University was psychoanalytic, following in the footsteps of Freud who reduced religion to an obsessional neurosis for the emotionally immature. Upon graduation, I began working as a psychologist in private practice. My patients have come to me often preoccupied with shame and failure, seeking symptom relief and personal happiness.

In my twenty years as a practicing psychologist, I felt that the soul was missing in the way I was taught to practice. The spirituality that guided the first half of my life was missing to a large degree. Thinking back on my life as a priest, I further observed, in agreement with Freud, that some used religion to satisfy a variety of emotional needs that were not always the healthiest. I have looked for ways to integrate healthy spirituality with emotional maturity. I have attempted to bring soul back into my work with my patients as an avenue to healing and growth. What I am discovering is that both my former parishioners and my current patients are really looking for the same thing. They feel broken and seek wholeness. This book is the fruit of my efforts to develop a psychology with soul and spirit.

HOW TO USE THIS BOOK

This book is divided into two parts. The first four chapters of part one describe what depression looks like, its similarity to addiction, how it develops, and how it shapes the personality. The second part presents an overview of the Twelve Steps and how each of the steps can be used as a practical guide to recovering from and growing through depression. Practices are offered as recovery aids. The case examples are composites of the stories of various patients, with details changed sufficiently to protect their confidentiality.

The Twelve Steps arose from a group experience. Bill Wilson consulted with many others, formed support groups, and refined the steps. The steps were formulated from the experience of alcoholics who gathered with a common goal, to become sober and improve their lives. They gathered in small groups to share their life experiences and work the steps. Within the fellowship they found support, understanding, and hope.

Suffering from depression, you tend to isolate yourself, which over time will only deepen your unhappiness. As the experience of the AA fellowship testifies, you cannot heal from your addiction to depression alone. You need the support and encouragement of others on this perilous journey. I recommend that you use this book, not alone, but with at least one companion. It may be a therapist, a spouse, a close friend, or another who also suffers depression. Freud observed that ultimately it is love that heals. You cannot love or be loved in isolation.

You may decide to join a support group. In your area you may find some depression support groups. You may seek out a group like Emotions Anonymous, which uses the Twelve Steps as a guide for working through various emotional struggles, including depression. Check out their website to see how the groups work and where they are located.

My dream is that groups will emerge that use the Twelve Steps specifically for recovery from depression. I would call them Depression Anonymous groups. You may feel inspired to gather a self-help group yourself. You are not alone in your suffering.

If you choose not to join with others, you can benefit from working with this book alone and using the exercises at the end of the chapters to aid in your own recovery. The Steps need to be worked, not just thought about. For personal transformation, they must become a daily practice.

Family members can also benefit from this book. They can come to understand and accept their own sense of powerlessness to overcome the mood addiction of their loved ones. Ironically, you may even find yourself becoming depressed caring for your depressed loved ones.

Mental health professionals who treat depressed patients may benefit from the book's presentation of a new way to think about depression and its treatment.

Clergy and religious authorities may appreciate the book's suggestions that spiritual practice can enhance psychological wellbeing. It may provide you with a new way of looking at spirituality, presented in contemporary, this-worldly language.

When depressed, you are preoccupied with a sense of loss, with what is missing. Your world narrows. Working the Steps will bring a surprising result, a renewed hope in life. The emptiness, the sense of scarcity, of your life will be transformed into a sense of abundance and gratitude. Your world expands. The awakening of your spirit will bring new life through an enlarged consciousness, as expressed in the Tao Te Ching (3):

> Be content with what you have;
> rejoice in the way things are.
> When you realize nothing is lacking,
> the whole world belongs to you (44).

My wish is that this book may aid you in uncovering the abundance already present in the midst of the ever-changing circumstances of your life. Living with gratitude is the way to a joyful life.

PART ONE
DEPRESSION AS AN ADDICTION

Dennis Ortman, Ph.D.

1

The Many Faces of Depression
Living With Loss

"So we live, forever saying farewell."

—Rilke

"Is the sadness you feel bitter or sweet? Is it a friend or a foe?" When you are in the depths of depression, hating yourself and your world, unable to motivate yourself for any activity, it is bitter. Depression is the enemy, a noonday demon you long to exorcise. However, as your recovery progresses, you will come to experience your sad mood, and all your painful feelings, as allies in your journey toward growth and maturity. When patients complain about how much pain they feel and beg me to show them a way out, I assure them, "Your pain shows that you are alive, not dead. Let's work to find the new life that's trying to break through the pain."

SADNESS, THE PAIN OF LIVING

Because we live in bodies which constantly change and interact with the world, we have feelings. We naturally have emotional reactions to what happens to us. Unpleasant experiences repulse us, moving us to withdraw to protect ourselves. Pleasant experiences energize us to seek more of what we desire. In our ever-changing world, we naturally feel joy as new life unfolds and sadness as the old and familiar passes away.

Our sadness and sorrow are natural reactions that serve survival purposes. In fact, they are signs of intelligence. Animals live by their instincts, only in the present moment. Because we are conscious, we humans are aware of the passage of time, alert to loss and gain. We are aware of changes around us and their consequences on our wellbeing, and so we make adjustments. Hardwired into our brains is a built-in threat protection and safety-seeking system. In the experience of loss, sadness prepares us to let go of the past and prepare for a new future.

When we feel sadness, sorrow, or grief, we tend to withdraw into ourselves for protection. We hibernate for a time to conserve our energies to adjust to the change. If we lose someone or something that is important to us, like a loved one, our job, or our self-esteem, we need to feel the pain before we can let go. Pain motivates the letting go.

In our sad mood, we become contemplatives who search for the meaning in the loss. We look for some larger perspective to make sense of it. Through this natural grieving process, we give up our personal investment in what passed and prepare to shift our energy to the new life that emerges. We come to accept the loss to free us for something new. That is the cycle of nature. Dying leads to new life. We consciously engage in this process through our painful, life-renewing grief.

If we embrace our sadness from this larger perspective, we can avoid becoming bitter at the inevitable losses in life. In fact, we gain wisdom that comes only from the suffering of loss. Our sadness makes us aware of the impermanence of life. Everything passes. Nothing remains. We learn to let go of what we cannot change, and we learn humility in the process. The pain of loss makes us release our attachment to persons and things we falsely believe will provide lasting happiness. In our pain, we also sense our deep longing for what can last. We search for some firm ground on which to stand in our free-fall life. We open our hearts to receive a gift of permanence we cannot create for ourselves.

Sadness also makes our hearts tender. If we manage to avoid self-pity, we realize that all of us are in the same boat. We all suffer the pain of countless losses and long for happiness. Sadness plants seeds of empathy and compassion in our hearts, enabling us to stand in the shoes of those who suffer. We appreciate more fully the tragic life we all share. This heartfelt awareness can further motivate us to help relieve suffering in the world, and not contribute to its pain.

Imagine a world without sadness or sorrow. Would it be heaven or hell? In your depressed mood, you imagine a paradise with unbounded bliss. But think again. To wish for such a world is avoidance of the real world of continual change, of loss and gain, of death and new life. Such a world would be static, without life. Change signals newness and life, but also includes loss. We feel sadness naturally at losing what we care for. Our sadness manifests what we hold dear. A world without sadness or sorrow would be a dead place without compassion. It would be a world without heart.

For many, the normal sadness, sorrow, and grief of life become a living hell. When the sad mood persists, deepens, and becomes overwhelming, you suffer clinical depression. The following are sketches of sadness in excess, called depressive disorders.

MAJOR DEPRESSIVE DISORDER

Paula, a middle-aged woman suffering emotional storms:

"Black moods seem to come out of nowhere and take me over. I heard them once called 'brain storms.' That describes what I feel perfectly. When the storm suddenly comes, there's a howling tempest in my brain. I can't focus on anything, can't think clearly, and can't make any decisions. I'm so agitated I can't sleep and have no en-

ergy or interest to do anything. I just want to curl up in a ball and die. These storms come unannounced, blow through me, and disappear after a couple of weeks. When it happens, I'm just plain miserable and intolerable to be around.

I was shy and withdrawn as a child. I really became depressed in my twenties, when I was first hospitalized for a suicide attempt. I understand where my depression came from. Almost everyone in my family has some degree of depression. My father withdrew when the moods overtook him, and my mother became mean and cruel. The only relief I find now between the depressive periods is smoking cigarettes, gardening, and caring for the dogs I foster from the animal shelter. I can identify with these outcast animals and want to help them."

Major depression comes like a sudden thunderstorm that completely incapacitates you. Sometimes you can identify triggers that announce it's coming, such as a loss of health, a death in the family, or a broken relationship. However, most often, the storms come out of the blue. Some change in your brain chemistry precipitates a cascading series of events. Joy disappears from your life, replaced by despair and hopelessness. Your mind is in a fog, and your body shuts down. You have no interest or pleasure in your life. You cannot eat or sleep as you did before. Thoughts of death fill your mind.

These storms do not really come from nowhere. Research shows that we inherit a predisposition to mood disorders from our family. Given the tendency to blame both yourself and others, you may blame your parents for your illness and yourself for being weak. Many of my patients complain of guilt for passing on their genes to their children, feeling responsible for their mental problems. But is that fair? Who chooses their own genetic makeup?

PSYCHOTIC DEPRESSION

Jennifer, a suicidal woman with two children:

"I've never been happy in my marriage. The only good thing that has come of it is my two children. My husband is a drunk. When he drinks he becomes mean. When I argue with him, he can become violent. I can't believe I was so stupid to marry someone just like my father. That depresses me. After fighting with my husband, I often feel hopeless and trapped and fall into a deep depression. I'm inconsolable at those times and just want to sleep. I have zero energy. I literally can't do anything. My sister has to come and take care of the children when I get that way. I feel so guilty about that, but can't help myself.

One time I became so depressed that I didn't want to live anymore. I began making plans about how I would kill myself. I didn't want to leave my children with my alcoholic husband, so I also thought about how I would kill them. I believed we would all be better off dead. That was a crazy idea. I felt so desperate I didn't know what else to do. One day the news covered the story of a woman who murdered her children. That shocking story woke me up. I realized how delusional I had become. That motivated me finally to get help."

In the depths of depression, you feel dead inside. You begin to focus all the rage you feel at the unfairness of your life on yourself. Violent thoughts preoccupy you, thoughts of turning all that aggression against yourself. Of course, the most violent act is to kill yourself. Such thinking can become delusional, out of touch with reality. You imagine destroying the world by eliminating yourself. Thoughts of how sad others would be at your demise fill your mind. In reality, you seek revenge through your death. You fantasize transforming your miserable life into a peaceful one through death. Your suicidal wish expresses a desperate desire for instant self-transformation. It is a desire for a quick fix. But in reality, suicide closes off the possibility of new life.

PERSISTENT DEPRESSIVE DISORDER

Alice, a woman feeling cheated by life:

"I've been jinxed. Nothing has ever gone right for me. It began in childhood. I was the fat kid everyone picked on. In high school, no boys ever wanted to date me. And then there's my health. I've suffered from asthma my whole life and had several auto accidents in which I was severely injured. I tried to make up for all my failures by being good at my job. I became an extremely competent executive secretary, a perfectionist. I took pride in my work. Would you believe I was fired because I complained so much about problems in the company? I just wanted the business to succeed. Even now, I'm the one who has to take care of our elderly parents because my siblings don't want to have anything to do with them. You'd think my parents would appreciate all my help, but they just take me for granted.

I often stay awake at night thinking about all the unfair things that happened to me. I also worry about the future. I don't know if I'll ever find a job that suits me and my abilities. I've had so many failures dating, I don't believe I'll ever find the right man and get married."

Carl, a man who could not say no to anyone:

"I've tried to please people my whole life. As a child, I wanted to please my parents and teachers. When I was married, I wanted to please my wife and my kids. At work, my bosses and coworkers. I never said 'no' to my friends when they asked for help. When anyone asked me to do something, I always said 'yes' immediately without out thinking. But afterward, I often regretted agreeing because I really didn't want to do it. So my whole life I did what others asked of me and came to hate myself for being a people-pleaser. I wanted people to like me, but ended up not liking myself."

Your feelings follow your thoughts. As you think, so you feel. When negative thoughts of failure and defeat fill your mind, you become depressed. The habit of negative thinking can develop early in life and result in a persistent depressive disorder. It used to be called dysthymia, which means, "lacking strong feeling," a loss of passion in life. The severity of this depression is not quite like that of major depression, but it still drains you of happiness.

You are your own worst enemy. Actually, that is good news because you can change the way you think. Typically, when you are depressed you develop unrealistic expectations about the world and your life. You can become a perfectionist in your thinking. I often ask my depressed patients, "What do you think the odds are of you being perfect?" They respond, "Not very good." "In fact, it's zero," I point out. If you expect perfection, you will always feel disappointed in your life and in yourself. The result is low self-esteem. At war within yourself, you engage in battles you can never win.

COMPLICATED GRIEF

Margaret, a woman who grieved the loss of her husband:

"I married the love of my life, and we were together for forty years. We did everything together, had three children, built a beautiful home, and ran a business. I can't tell you how devastated I was when John died suddenly of a heart attack. I wasn't prepared for it. At first, I went into shock. I couldn't believe he was gone. Then, I became angry at being abandoned by him, left with a home and business to run. Then, the depression set in and took hold of my life. I couldn't sleep. Some days I spent hours crying. I felt so overwhelmed and helpless taking care of our large home and business. I felt so lost. John handled all the financial affairs. I always thought of myself as an independent woman and now realized how dependent I was on him.

It's been three years since he died. I still feel lost without him. The crying spells are less frequent now, but I can't stop thinking about him and our life together. I'm so impatient with myself that I can't get over the grief. What's wrong with me? We used to drink together to relax after work. Now I find myself drinking more, often more than is good for me. I'm afraid I'm developing a problem, but feel too ashamed to seek help."

Depression is a reaction to loss. The more important the loss, such as a spouse, the deeper the depression. A period of grief is natural after the death of a loved one. In the grieving process, you work through the feelings of loss and come to an acceptance of a new life without the loved one. Grief frees you to love again. However, if there were unresolved issues in your life or relationship, the grief becomes complicated. Full acceptance of the loss will occur only after the underlying unresolved feelings, such as anger and guilt, are worked through.

When depressed, there is a danger of self-medicating with alcohol or other drugs. Research indicates that nearly a third (32%) of those who suffer a mood disorder also abuse substances (1). You imagine that the alcohol or drugs will provide relief. However, using them only makes your depression worse. Alcohol is a depressant that will deepen your depression and neutralize your medication. If you drink enough, you risk becoming addicted and then have a second problem.

CHILDHOOD TRAUMA

Carol, a woman carrying shame from her childhood:

"In therapy I had a flashback of being molested at a very young age. There was no one to protect me. My father worked long hours, and my mother was depressed. When she wasn't withdrawn, she became a bitch, constantly criticizing me. I remember being desperately unhappy growing up. Because my parents were so absent, as the oldest, I took care of my younger brothers and sisters. I hated the job and looked for a way to escape. I did that by becoming pregnant and leaving home at seventeen. But that was a huge mistake. My boyfriend left me alone to care for our child. Again, I was thrust into a role I hated.

Now these many years later, I'm still unhappy. My daughter is grown. I live alone and fear controls my life. I recently retired from a job I loved. Now I never leave my messy house. In fact, it is more than messy. It's a disaster. For years I've hoarded things. Junk is piled from floor to ceiling. I'm too embarrassed to invite anyone into my home, so I live as a hermit. My self-imposed job now is to clean the place out. Every time I get started, my stomach gets in a knot. My throat tightens and my teeth clench. I stop and distract myself on the computer. I'm really terrified what I might discover under all the accumulated stuff."

The past is never dead. It continues to live through you. If you have been traumatized in childhood by abuse or neglect, you will carry the scars for the rest of your life. The wounds may heal, but the residue of sadness and fear will remain. Events in later life will trigger flashbacks of your painful childhood. Unconsciously, you will recreate in your relationships unhealthy patterns you experienced in your family. Again, you will feel like a helpless victim. You repeat the past not to torment yourself, but to make it end differently.

Depression and anxiety work hand-in-hand. Depressed, you become preoccupied with the painful losses from your past. The losses of childhood are the most enduring because you were too helpless then to protect yourself. Anxious, you fear the losses of the past will continue into the future. You come to believe that only pain and suffering await you. To protect yourself, you withdraw into safe roles and routines. Your life shrinks, and your depression increases. You sense how much of your life remains unlived.

MIDLIFE CRISIS

Jim, facing middle-age disillusionment:

"My life has been perfect. I'm happily married to a beautiful, loving woman and have three wonderful children. I pursued the career of my dreams and have a comfortable lifestyle. I work hard and have been rewarded for my effort. Our home is in a fashionable neighborhood. Our kids attend the best schools, and they are doing well. I have all the toys. As I look around, I wouldn't exchange my life for anyone. I have arrived.

Yet I feel sad inside. As I look at my life, I have no reason to be sad. I'm probably the envy of my friends. Somehow, the excitement has left me. I feel bored. I keep going to work, but I have no enthusiasm for my job. Everything I do for my family and around the house has become a burden. There is no joy. What's the matter with me? Sometimes I think I'm just a spoiled child who has it all but is still dissatisfied."

Your depressed mood can spring from unidentified sources. In the midst of a happy life, discontent suddenly arises. It can leave you confused and feeling lost. However, if you view your life from a larger perspective, you recognize milestones, times of significant transition. Leaving home, getting married, having children, going through divorce, and the deaths of parents are such milestones. These transitions remind you of the impermanence of life. Everything arises and passes away so something new can be born.

Reaching middle age, with its gathering sense of mortality, is another major life passage. The depression you feel at that time is a message that some new life is pressing to be acknowledged. The disillusionment of dreams achieved beckons you to look more deeply at your life to search for what really lasts. The subtle aches and pains you feel remind you that death is on the horizon. That awareness makes you look inward to find what is of ultimate importance to you.

ADJUSTMENT DISORDER

Neil, a young man who lost his job:

"I was stunned when my boss called me into his office to tell me he was letting me go. It was my first job. I had worked there as an engineer for eight years and imagined making a career at that large company. I was in shock when I went home and told my wife. That night I couldn't sleep. In fact, I had a couple weeks of sleepless nights. I worried about so many things. How are we going to pay the bills? Will we lose the house? Will I ever find another job? And then the depression set in. I loved working there. My sense of security was lost. I missed all the friends I made. The anger simmered beneath the surface and erupted when I thought about the unfairness of laying me off. I was one of their best workers.

Through all the emotional upheaval, I began to make plans for finding another job. I saw it as my full-time job now. I knew I had skills others would want. So I redid my resume and posted it online. I searched the Internet and followed up on job leads. I contacted my friends in the field and let them know I was looking. As I became more active, I noticed that my mood lifted. And I didn't feel so frightened and angry. I knew this could be a new start."

Life is a merry-go-round of alternating loss and gain, failure and success, pain and joy. You must constantly adjust to changes, the new replacing the old. With your inborn sensitivity to the threat of loss, in the midst of change you become naturally preoccupied with the loss of the comfortably familiar. The potential gain fades into the background. For a period of time you mourn the loss and gather your energy to embark on a new path. Feelings of sadness, anger, and fear arise. You are not yourself in the painful adjustment period, which can become full-blown depression if you become stuck.

Most hate change because it creates uncertainty. It is a leap into the unknown. However, the pain of change stimulates growth. It motivates you to action. If you stay in the secure past, you will stagnate. The sameness will eventually kill your spirit. Changing circumstances awaken you to the possibility of new life. Accepting the loss of security and facing your fear of the unknown opens your heart and makes you strong. As the song goes, "If it does not kill you, it will make you strong."

BIPOLAR DISORDER

David, a man with manic episodes:

"I can be moody. But mostly I'm depressed. Almost anything can affect my mood, any disappointment, an argument with my wife, even a change in the weather. It doesn't take much to put me in a tailspin. Sometimes I just become irritable, everything bothers me. At other times, when the depression grabs me, I just want to be alone and do nothing. I want to sleep, but feel too restless to relax. Nothing gives me any satisfaction.

Every now and then, for some unknown reason, I feel energized, on top of the world. I can't sleep, but I don't care because I feel so motivated to keep working at my chores and hobbies. One time, after a healing service at church, I thought I was cured of my manic-depression and quit taking my medication. I was flying high for weeks. I was caught up in a whirlwind, and nothing could stop me. Ideas raced through my mind and I talked nonstop. I couldn't sleep for days, but it didn't matter because there was so much I wanted to do. I spoke my mind and told my wife off, like I always wanted. I thought I was Superman. I loved it—until I crashed. I fell into the blackest pit ever. Only being hospitalized and getting back on the medication saved my life."

Mood disorders are of two types: unipolar, which is just depression without the high, and bipolar, which alternates between highs and lows. When you are depressed, your system shuts down. You feel as if you have been drugged with a sedative-hypnotic. You sleepwalk through life in an agitated state. When you have bipolar disorder, previously called manic-depression, uncontrollable moods take over your life. Your moods fluctuate between lows and highs, in either rapid or slow succession. When low, you lack energy and motivation to engage in life. When high, you are energized as if you are on a stimulant drug. You cannot relax, sleep, or slow down the racing thoughts or pressured speech. Driven by grandiose ideas, you engage in erratic, and sometimes dangerous, behavior.

A MANY-COLORED TAPESTRY

Depression is not a seamless black cloth, the same for everybody suffering this illness. When patients come seeking relief, we investigate closely the exact nature of their mood together. We look at what it feels like, when it began, and how it unfolds in their lives.

Each depression is unique, a many-colored tapestry that is different for each person. Some painful moods are more severe than others, like the major depression of Paula and Jennifer, and the passing mood of Neil, composed of various shades of grey threads. The condition can be chronic, passing, or in repeating waves. The red strands of biology, a chemical imbalance, or genetic influence may stand out, as in the case of Paula who came from a family with a long history of mood disturbances. The black thread of psychotic thinking in self-loathing and paranoid ideas may appear. The exploding yellow of mania, as in the case of David, may show itself. The blue threads of life circumstances, involving mostly painful experiences of loss, may dominate the picture. Stubborn grief over these losses may darken the picture, as it did for Margaret. Some losses occur early in life, from childhood traumas suffered, as with Carol. The purple threads of trauma may weave through the entire tapestry, coloring the experiences into adulthood. Green strands that reflect temperament and unresolved inner conflicts, as in the cases of Alice and Carl, may be most noticeable. As with Jim, the orange threads of life transitions, the natural passages, may shape the portrait. The result of the weaving of these many threads is a colorful tapestry.

Healing and growth will come as you become acquainted with the unique tapestry of your life and moods. It may be hard to believe, but this tapestry has its own beauty, like no other. It displays the magnificence of your soul. It represents your gift to the world. Your life task will be to understand and appreciate all the colorful strands, work to untie the knots, and let the beauty show.

Dennis Ortman, Ph.D.

2

Depression as a Mood Addiction
Trying to Control the Uncontrollable

"God breaks the heart again and again
and again until it stays open."

—Hazrat Inayat Khan

There is no such thing as a happy drunk. Despite the portrayal of the carefree, happy-go-lucky drinker, such as a character from the TV show "Cheers," when an addiction takes hold, that person is miserable. He no longer drinks for pleasure. He drinks simply to feel normal. Even though he denies a problem, at some level he knows the harm his drinking causes himself and others. But he feels powerless to stop it, and so shame, guilt, and depression add to his woes.

Everyone has the blues from time to time. However, when a full-blown depression descends, you cannot escape the black cloud. You feel desperate and plea to anyone who will hear, "Please, help me get rid of the pain." You may make the rounds to friends and family who offer cliché-like advice, "Just push yourself...Be patient, and it will go away...Keep a positive attitude." Their suggestions drive you insane. You may see psychiatrists who offer a variety of medications and psychologists who explore your past or try to change your thinking. But the mood still may not lift. Its stubbornness frustrates you to no end.

In your sense of powerlessness, you understand the experience of an alcoholic. Your depressed mood has become your drug, although it offers no pleasure. Unfortunately, in its persistence, it may become the new normal for you.

Your futile efforts to control the uncontrollable and to get relief from your mood multiply your suffering. Not only do you feel the pain of the black mood, but you become depressed about being depressed. You hate your mood and feel helpless to do anything about it.

The experience of depression parallels that of addiction to alcohol and other drugs. The following are characteristics of both depression and addiction:

- Bittersweet excess.
- Denial, ignoring the obvious.
- Going in circles.
- Loss of control.
- Will to power, and defeat.
- Self-medicating the pain of life.
- Beyond cure.

Let me briefly explain how the experience of the alcoholic, as an example of an addicted person, overlaps with what you experience with depression.

BITTERSWEET EXCESS

"What's wrong with enjoying a drink every now and then?" Nothing, if it does not cause problems. Drinking with friends is a normal pleasure for many people. Alcohol helps them relax, let down their hair, and talk freely in social situations. It is a natural tranquilizer used as a social lubricant. Drinking has become so much a part of our culture that the effort to stop it during the Prohibition failed. "We want our beer!" placards were carried by protesters in a picture from an anti-Prohibition rally I saw recently.

Social drinking presents no problems until it increases, often imperceptibly, and crosses an invisible line to becoming alcoholic drinking. The reasons for consuming alcohol, often unconscious, shift from drinking for pleasure to drinking to feel normal. Alcoholics then want to drink to avoid the hangovers and shakes. They need to drink more and more just to feel normal. They manufacture excuses for their need to drink. At this point, the AA slogan applies, "One drink is too much, and a thousand is not enough."

Rachel, recounting the progression of her depression:

"I was a quiet, sensitive child. I spent many hours alone, lost in my imagination. As a teen, I wore black and hung around with a bunch of artist types. People called me Gothic. I didn't mind the label back then, and even took pride in it. I had a romantic spirit and became an English major in college. I loved to write poetry about lost love and death. Keats and Shelly were my favorites. But in my twenties, a black mood took over my life. I had no energy, hated my life, and just wanted to die. Thank God the storm lifted after a few months with medication. But it has come back several times with increasing ferocity, and I hang on by my fingertips just to survive."

Shakespeare's Juliet, enthralled with her love of Romeo, chanted, "Parting is such sweet sorrow." The brief sadness of separation only increases the joy of anticipating reunion with the beloved. Sadness is natural when separation and loss occur. The feelings of loss remove you from your head and bring you to your heart. Tenderness and compassion arise. A delicious tragic and romantic spirit may follow. Sorrow, although often bitter, can be sweet when you have hope for the future, for something new and exciting on the horizon.

The sweetness of sadness may sour, however, leaving only a bitter taste in your mouth. The natural experience of mourning a loss may intensify into a black mood that will not lift. Your body, mind, and spirit seem to die. In the grip of depression, you cannot eat or sleep normally. Sapped of energy, you cannot engage in life. Your agitated mind ruminates about past hurts and regrets. Thoughts of doom and gloom occupy your mind. Despair grips you. Feeling hopeless, you lose your will to live. You feel more dead than alive. Only the pain reminds you that there is still life in you.

Both addictive and mood disorders are marked by excess. They may begin with a taste of sweetness, but soon shift to complete bitterness in their excess. While alcoholics drink more than others, those suffering mood disorders experience more intense and prolonged sadness than the average person. Both reach a point in their excess that the pain is barely tolerable. They only want relief from the pain. Paradoxically, embracing that pain can move them to seek help, and eventually recovery.

DENIAL, IGNORING THE OBVIOUS

Alcoholics live in denial about their drinking, which allows the chaos and confusion to continue. They suffer from a disease of perception. They cannot add correctly, insisting that they had only "a couple drinks," while their loved ones come to a different total. Their memory is selective. Alcoholics seem to remember only the good times drinking and forget the hangovers and their obnoxious behavior while drunk. They recall the drink, and not the drunk. They are also masters at rationalizing. Alcoholics can give you a million reasons why they need to drink, saying with complete conviction, "I drink because I'm happy, sad, stressed, or just enjoy the taste." In their selective awareness, they overlook the obvious harm they cause themselves and others.

The consequences of the denial can be catastrophic. Drunkenness leads to accidents, failed marriages, lost jobs, and premature death. It allows the illness to progress and go untreated. The result, as AA puts it bluntly, is "insanity or death."

Katherine, complaining of health problems:

> *"I went to see my doctor because I'd been feeling bad for a long time. I felt so tired and just wanted to sleep all day. My stomach was often upset for no reason, and I didn't want to eat. I had headaches that wouldn't go away and often felt dizzy. I had too many aches and pains to count. Well, my doctor listened patiently as I told him about my woes. So he ran a battery of tests. The next week he called me into his office and said, 'Katherine, all the tests did not indicate any medical cause for your symptoms. I think you may be depressed.' I was stunned by what he said and didn't believe it. I told him I was going for another opinion."*

You may not recognize that you are depressed because it is masked by so many physical symptoms. Depression takes over your body. You may believe you have a medical problem and check it out with your doctor, like many others. In fact, eighty percent of those diagnosed as depressed receive the diagnosis from their primary care physicians, not from mental health specialists. Tragically, only half of those who are depressed and go to their doctors with somatic complaints are correctly diagnosed with depression. It's estimated that only one in ten of those who are clinically depressed receive treatment. And their suffering continues.

Who wants to admit that they see a psychiatrist or psychologist? There is such a stigma regarding mental illness in our society that you may feel ashamed that you suffer from depression. In their ignorance, people think, "You are just weak…You can get over it if you want…What did you do to cause it?" The prejudice against mental problems may keep you from acknowledging your depression and getting help. The results of your denial may be just as catastrophic as that of any addiction, insanity or death by suicide.

Both the addicted and the depressed ignore the warning signs from their bodies, their families, and their friends who know they have a problem. They suffer from a case of distorted perception. Their sense of shame keeps them in denial. Tragically, their denial will prolong the suffering unnecessarily. It will keep them from getting help for conditions that are very treatable.

GOING IN CIRCLES

Alcoholics are stuck in "stinking thinking" and in their behavior. They develop many strange ideas about alcohol, such as, "I can't live without it." They come to believe that they will find happiness in a bottle, that drinking will magically erase all their problems, at least for the moment. They think they need to drink when they are happy, sad, anxious, or angry. In other words, whenever they feel anything. Their awareness becomes suspiciously selective. They remember only the good times drinking, with a "euphoric recall," and forget the trouble it caused. Their preoccupation is the next drink.

The obsessive thinking spills over into compulsive behaviors. Alcoholics develop bizarre rituals, rules, and routines around drinking. They proclaim with unblinking assurance that they cannot be an alcoholic because they never drink alone, in the morning, all day, or every day. They begin to plan their days and social activities around alcohol consumption. They choose friends who drink just like them. Soon, without realizing it, alcohol becomes the organizing principle of their lives. It is their constant companion, and eventually, their only friend.

John, consumed with grief:

"My wife of forty years died a year ago. I can't stop thinking about her. When she was alive, we did everything together. She was my soul mate. I keep thinking about all the good times we had, all the vacations and the holidays with the family. And now she's gone. My kids are concerned about me and plead, 'Dad, you have to move on with your life.' But I'm old and feel like my life is over. I'm just waiting to die and wish I wouldn't wake up in the morning. All I do is dwell on the past. I don't feel like doing anything. I stay home. I don't want to see anyone. I just want to be left alone with my memories."

When you are depressed, your mind goes in circles. The center of that circle is the past. More specifically, what you miss from the past. You are preoccupied with a sense of loss. It might be nostalgia about what was and is no more. Or it might be all the regrets. You ruminate about "what could have been" and all the "if onlys." If you recall wonderful events that happened in your life, you do not allow yourself to savor them. Instead, you remind yourself that the good times are now over. Your mind is in a rut, dwelling on what is now missing. It is as if your mind is a radio tuned to one station, the sad music of loss.

Your preoccupation with all the losses and the past prevents you from living in the present. Compulsively, you avoid engaging fully in the present moment. Since all is lost, there is no reason to live. So you withdraw into your own world of negative notions. You isolate yourself, avoiding the companionship of those who can make you feel alive. Wishing to be dead, you live as if you already are.

Both the depressed and the addicted go in circles with their minds and their behavior. Alcoholics obsess about the next drink, while the depressed dwell on painful losses from the past. Alcoholics develop rituals and routines, chasing the party for their next drink. Those who are depressed become lost in their negative thoughts, isolate themselves, and withdraw from life. They remain stuck until they fall on their faces onto the path of recovery.

LOSS OF CONTROL

What makes someone an alcoholic is not how much or how often she drinks, but what happens when she drinks. The primary symptom is loss of control. When she drinks, she is not sure when she will stop. She may not lose control every time, but as the illness progresses she becomes intoxicated more often. Because of her denial, she may believe she can stop whenever she likes. However, in her stubbornness, she ignores all the evidence to the contrary. She will only enter recovery when she fully acknowledges the reality, her powerlessness over alcohol.

As the illness progresses, the loss of control, with its devastating effects, deepens. The drinking takes over her life. An AA saying describes the decline so accurately: "First, the man takes the drink; then, the drink takes the drink; and finally, the drink takes the man."

Richard, feeling trapped in his job:

"After high school I wanted to go to college, but my girlfriend became pregnant. I had to find a good enough paying job to support the family. So I worked on the assembly line. I hated it, all the noise, grime, and boring routine. I'm not surprised I became depressed. I hated my life so much that I attempted suicide to escape. My family put me in the hospital where the doctors medicated me. Despite the medication and counseling, the depression descended on me regularly, and there was nothing I could do about it. I had suicidal thoughts, and the doctor increased my medication. All I could do was wait until the mood passed. I felt so helpless."

Another name for depression is "learned helplessness." When you feel trapped in a situation that you cannot escape, you may withdraw into a black mood. It is a sign that you feel trapped and helpless. You may also begin to think of yourself as a victim, persecuted by cruel fate and unable to defend yourself. Thinking like a victim then deepens your dark mood.

You may also feel victimized by the depression itself. Depressed, you feel like you have fallen into a black hole that sucks your life and energy. You cannot climb out of the pit. The more you try, the more you fall back into the abyss and feel defeated. Not only do you feel helpless confronting your life situation, but you have lost control of your mind and mood.

Like any addiction, the sense of lost control progresses: "First, the man is depressed; then, he is depressed about being depressed; and finally, the depression takes the man."

The core of both depression and addiction is the loss of control. At some level, both addicted and depressed individuals realize that they are under the influence of a power greater than themselves, but they feel powerless to disengage. Both see themselves as helpless victims in life. Acknowledging a spiritual Power greater than themselves provides an escape to new life.

WILL TO POWER, AND DEFEAT

Alcoholics Anonymous describes alcoholics as "self-centered in the extreme," and as those whose trouble is caused by "the misuse of willpower." Feeling so helpless and out of control in his life, the alcoholic craves power and control. When he first begins drinking, the alcoholic discovers the magical quality of alcohol to transform his moods and personality. He enjoys the pleasurable feeling of intoxication and escaping painful reality. With time and experience, he finds in alcohol the means to control his mind, mood, and world whenever he wants. Alcohol is his personal genie in a bottle.

For a time, alcohol is a wonder drug, the elixir of life—until the addiction takes hold. As his drinking increases, the miracle drug that freed him begins to control him. The instrument he used to master his world now enslaves him. That bitter truth is hard for the alcoholic to admit. He cannot tolerate the disillusionment and give up the drug he depends on. Instead, he redoubles his efforts to control his life, his drinking, and those around him. He blames others for his problems and attempts to change his drinking pattern. As his efforts at control inevitably fail, he feels defeated. His low self-esteem drives him to try harder to exercise power and control. He drinks more.

And the vicious, downward spiral continues.

Amanda, a self-proclaimed perfectionist:

"I'm a perfectionist. My mother drummed it into me, 'It's not worth doing unless you do it right.' That became my guide for living. I worked hard at my job as a nurse, holding myself and my coworkers to the highest standards. I always pushed myself at work and led by example. At home, I taught my children to behave honorably and properly. They grew up to be outstanding citizens and parents. But when my son got divorced, I went into a tailspin. I blamed myself, imagining I did something wrong. I worried about the children, the effect the divorce would have on them. I became deeply depressed, and then depressed about being depressed. For the first time in my life I felt I couldn't take care of myself. I've always dreaded being a burden to anyone."

If you are depressed, life has disappointed you. You feel a sense of loss because your hopes have been dashed in some way. You hoped for something more than your life delivered. Perhaps you expected better health, a more stable relationship, or a more satisfying job. When your expectations were not met, disappointment set in with an accompanying depressed mood. Feeling the losses so deeply, you became pessimistic about ever being happy again. Behind every pessimist is a hidden optimist, someone who had dreams that were not realized.

In your disappointment, you look for someone or something to blame. With your depressed mind, you end up blaming yourself and suffer a painful loss of self-esteem. You tell yourself, "I must have done something wrong." Then, you take it a step further, "Something is wrong with me." The anger at the loss is directed at yourself. Paradoxically, blaming yourself gives you the illusion of control. If circumstances or fate stole your happiness, then you cannot protect yourself or recover the loss. If you look to yourself as the cause of the problem, then you have some hope that you can create a different outcome the next time. In your all-or-none thinking, you wish for total control over your life by taking full responsibility for all your suffering.

Anger resides close to the surface in both addicted and depressed persons. A war rages within them. They are angry that they suffer so many losses and have so little control over their lives. To compensate, the alcoholic drinks to make the world go away. The depressed persons direct all their aggression against themselves. They risk taking the ultimate power move in killing themselves as revenge for not getting what they want from life. Surrendering the need for control becomes the only way to win the battle.

SELF MEDICATING THE PAIN OF LIFE

Alcoholism arises from suffering and is a means to relieve suffering. Most alcoholics, contrary to popular belief, are sensitive souls searching for something more in life. They know from bitter experience that life is hard and look for some way to make it easier.

Imagine the joy when drinkers discover in alcohol a power greater than themselves to relieve them of their suffering and give them some momentary pleasure. They find in alcohol a medicine that acts more quickly, simply, and effectively than anything else they have tried. Alcohol is their natural, easily accessible tranquilizer that numbs the pain of life. It offers a quick fix, a magical cure. It eliminates the need to work at developing coping skills, which require so much time and effort.

Drinking offers another benefit. It allows them to withdraw from the hassles of life. When drinking, they are carefree and do not have a worry in the world. The nagging wife, the boring job, and the screaming kids can be forgotten in the moments of sweet intoxication. Responsibilities are put on the back burner, perhaps put off indefinitely. The alcoholic justifies his drinking bout, saying, "Everyone needs a break every now and then."

Stanley, a man caught up in nostalgia:

> *"My wife complains that I live more in the past than the present. She's probably right. I'm a nostalgic person, often thinking about how my life could have been different. I have so many regrets. I can't help blaming myself for all the mistakes I made in my life. I know it makes me sad, but I do it anyway. I think I learned that way of thinking from my father. He was a tragic figure, a refugee from Poland who felt trapped in a factory job he hated. He longed for the old country and never*

seemed to be at home here. My father spent many hours alone taking long walks. I missed him. In some ways I felt like I never had a father."

When in a black mood, your mind becomes preoccupied with the past and with loss. Upon closer examination, your depression is a resistance to the natural flow of life. Life is continual change, with inevitable losses and gains. You lament the losses and overlook any anticipated gains. What may not be apparent is that what you think you are sad about may disguise a deeper trauma that you are unable to face. You may have been abused as a child, been abandoned by a parent, or suffered a devastating illness. Allowing yourself to feel the pain of those deeper losses may be too overwhelming. Your sad mood, as painful as that is, may sedate you in your woundedness.

Your dark mood causes you to withdraw from life and all its overwhelming responsibilities. Your depression may be a refuge in difficult times. You build a wall around yourself. Your lack of energy and motivation keep you from venturing out of your self-created enclosure. You display a "keep away" sign. Your preoccupation with regrets and self-criticism excludes thinking about other matters. Protected by a wall of sadness, you disengage from life.

"Avoidance" is the middle name of both addicted and depressed persons. Both are exquisitely sensitive people who have difficulty coping with life. Their drinking or mood may disguise deep hurts. Easily overwhelmed, they develop survival strategies to maintain their wellbeing. They find relief from the unavoidable pain of life by numbing themselves with a drug or by withdrawing into their sorrows. But the pain inevitably breaks through, extending an invitation to recovery.

BEYOND CURE

Many alcoholics entertain a persistent fantasy that one day they will be able to drink like everyone else. Alcoholics Anonymous bursts their bubble, proclaiming, "Once an alcoholic, always an alcoholic." The program suggests that alcoholics have an allergy to alcohol and a disease for which there is no cure. However, there is a simple solution to the immediate problem: do not take a drink. "It's only the first drink you have to worry about," AA reminds it members.

It may take a while for an alcoholic to accept the reality of their condition. It usually takes many failed attempts at social drinking, several relapses, and a world of trouble before they accept the truth and admit, "I have an incurable illness called alcoholism." That awareness frees them from the hopeless struggle to control their drinking. It also makes them vigilant about their vulnerability to relapse.

A second awareness dawns on them if they accept their condition as chronic. Initially, they thought drinking was the problem. All they had to do was quit drinking, and then they would be happy. Through recovery they learn that their drinking is a symptom of a deeper problem they ignore. Self-centeredness and character defects are at the root of their excessive drinking and consequent misery. They need to make major lifestyle changes to find a lasting happiness. Their challenge, then, is not merely to remain sober, but to have a quality sobriety, a wholesome, enriched life. That requires a lifetime of effort. Alcoholics remain hopeless about a cure, but hopeful about recovering a life worth living.

Susan, an elderly woman who battled depression her whole life:

"I've had bouts of depression my whole life. I was first hospitalized as a teenager. After a breakup with my boyfriend, I attempted suicide. It seems the black cloud never left me after that. I had periods when the sadness lifted briefly, but it always came back, sometimes with a vengeance. There were periods when I felt so miserable that I only wanted to die. I've been hospitalized several times for suicide attempts. The doctors have prescribed every new medication that hit the market. It worked for a while, and then the depression returned. I've been in counseling off-and-on for years, read all the self-help books, and even had shock treatments. But the depression persisted. I don't feel hopeless after all these years, just resigned. I accept my identity as a depressed person and offer it up to God."

For many, the depressed mood comes and goes as you adjust to the many changes in your life. However, for some, the black cloud never completely dissipates. It enshrouds you again and again, with a tormenting regularity. The doctors tell you that you have a chemical imbalance, a genetic predisposition toward depression. Or you may have had such traumatic experiences in childhood, or later, that the scars never heal. You have an extreme sensitivity to loss, which is activated by the ever-changing events of your life. It may take a lifetime of effort to avoid being overcome by your condition. Like the alcoholic, resigning to the reality of your condition can propel you to a deeper spiritual search for meaning and an enriched life.

Depression, like an addiction, can take control of your life and not let go. One elderly woman lamented to me, "I've been so sad my whole life, I wouldn't recognize happiness if it hit me in the face." Clearly, the roots of depression and addiction are deep and grow from a common soil.

Dennis Ortman, Ph.D.

3

The Process of Addiction
Contending with Waves Of Loss

"Every particle of creation sings its own song of what is and what is not.
Hearing what is can make you wise;
hearing what is not can drive you crazy."

— Ghalib

Both the addicted and the depressed find themselves drowning in emotional high seas. They desperately struggle to ride the waves, but can barely keep themselves afloat. Too often they sink. Those deep waters that engulf them are fed by a variety of streams. Some streams flow as a trickle, while others come as a torrent. Dark waters mingle, creating a bottomless, black sea. Natural, biological, temperamental, and cultural streams fill that watery place.

What streams flow into the pool of addiction and depression?

- The natural experience of loss and longing.

- A brain exquisitely sensitive to loss.

- A melancholic temperament bent toward the negative.

- Society's great expectations, fueling our longings and disappointments.

THE NATURAL STREAM: LOSS AND LONGING

Miriam, a lifetime of losses:

"My mother died ten years ago. Not a day goes by that I don't think about her. Sometimes, even after all these years, I suddenly break into tears because I miss her so much. What's the matter with me? As much as I loved my mother, I also hated her. After my father abandoned the family, my mother fell into a deep depression. She leaned on me, her only daughter, to take care of her. She could be mean and demanding, a cruel tyrant. I felt like her slave. My whole life I've been looking to be loved. That's not asking for much. I married a man who was self-centered and cared only about himself. He died, leaving me penniless. Now I work at a job I hate, just to keep my head above water. I feel like I'm drowning."

Life begins and ends with loss. When we are born, we lose the comfort and security of the womb. Physically separated from our mother' body, we are cast into a new world and begin to breathe on our own. At death, we are physically torn away from our familiar world, losing everyone and everything we care for. In between, we adjust to constant change as life presents countless, often unanticipated, challenges. We choose a course. Each decision we make then creates new challenges.

Those depressed and those addicted have generally suffered a disproportionate number of painful losses in their lives. Many suffered abuse and neglect as children, feeling overwhelmed or abandoned. The losses mount up. Throughout their lives, they experience the death of loved ones, breakdowns of health, or heart-wrenching disappointments. An estimated ninety percent of those addicted to drugs have been traumatized in some way, suffering overwhelming hurt. Depression also disguises deep wounds of deprivation.

Caught up in all the comings and goings, we may realize that a gain accompanies every loss. Every ending announces a new beginning. In fact, the ceaseless change is a sign of life, of new life being born through the dying of the old. The only constant we can count on is ongoing change. That fact both thrills and terrifies us because it continually moves us from familiar territory into the unknown future.

Mixed with the continuous sense of loss are deep longings for a fixed point in our turning world. In the midst of our experience of confusion and chaos, we long for certainty, security, and stability. We long for something permanent that we can hold on to. We long for some firm ground on which we can stand in the swirl of life. Feeling homeless and unprotected, we desire a comfortable place to reside. So our hearts are torn. We live in a world we experience as riotous, vital, and confusing, yet we want security, comfort, and predictability. We want to return to the cozy warmth of the womb.

How do we cope with this inner conflict, embracing both life-giving change and our desire for permanence at the same time? How do we face an unknown future? How do we relax with the mystery of it all? We have two choices. We can surrender to the mystery of our unfolding lives and grow. Or we can regress into a childlike obsession with security.

When depressed, we refuse to surrender and grow. Seeking security, we hang on desperately to some illusionary life preserver in our personal sea of change. We resist the natural flow of our life and develop some fixed ideas to give us an imaginary stability. What are some of these fixed ideas? We focus on the past, our losses, and all our hurts. We think of ourselves as helpless victims. We entertain impossible standards and lament what is missing in our lives. We blame ourselves for all that has gone wrong in our lives. In the midst of our chaotic lives, we proclaim, "This I know to be true. It gives me a sense of certainty." What we avoid is fully engaging ourselves in our current life.

Those addicted to drugs also rebel against life as it is. They resist becoming active participants in their daily lives by using their drug of choice. They become stuck in their thinking and behavior. Like the depressed, they think poorly of themselves, indulge in self-blame, and consider themselves victims of a cruel life. They use their drug to self-medicate painful losses and believe they can find happiness in getting high. Their drug-induced utopia is really an escape from the flow of life.

THE BIOLOGICAL STREAM: A SENSITIVE BRAIN

In the midst of this topsy-turvy world, are we destined to be depressed? Are some born to be depressed? The answer is "yes and no." As science comes to understand the complex workings of the brain, we realize how much we have in common with the animal world. Not only our bodies, but our brains have evolved along pathways whose origins reach back into the animal kingdom. We are the growing edge of that kingdom. Our brains are designed to react to change, loss, and threat like our mammalian ancestors.

What has been called the "old brain" has been inherited from our evolutionary history. More specifically, the way we regulate our affects in adapting to our changing world is conditioned by the systems of the emotional brain. Three common patterns, all contributing to our survival, have been identified (1). The first is the threat protection and safety-seeking system. We live in a world of danger where we must fight for our survival. As Darwin demonstrated, only the fittest survive. This system detects threats, activates protective emotions, and initiates self-defensive actions. When a threat is detected, the amygdala, the small almond-shaped fear center in the brain, is activated, causing the stress hormone cortisol to be released. We react emotionally, with anger, anxiety, or disgust, and behaviorally, by fighting, fleeing, or freezing. The stress response affects our concentration, memory, and sensitivity to further threat. Our depressed mood is a threat protection response in the face of the loss of what is important to us.

The second is the activating, energizing system, which enables us to seek out the good things in life. It moves us to make efforts toward achievement and acquisition, satisfying our desires. When this system is activated, we feel excited, vital, and motivated. We feel alive and engage in fulfilling activities. Dopamine, noradrenalin, and serotonin, which are chemical messengers, bathe the brain. These neurotransmitters affect appetite, sleep, and motivation. This system can become exhausted by overwork, stress, and prolonged negative thinking. Depression tones down the activity of this brain system, making us more passive.

The third system regulates the experience of being soothed and content. Endorphins, the body's natural opiates, and the hormone oxytocin are released throughout the body. Their release creates feelings of calm and wellbeing without intentional striving. In stressful situations, we feel soothed and peaceful. When relating to others, we feel warmth, affection, and kindness. These feelings move us to become more social and to connect with others. Depression inhibits the activity of this system, causing a loss of joy and desire to socialize.

Over the past two million years, the human brain has evolved beyond that of the animals, resulting in a "new brain" in the frontal cortex. We have the ability to think, imagine, predict, and plan. Our logical brains enable us to be creative in adjusting to the demands of our changing world. Beyond the instinctive reactions of our emotional brains, we can respond freely to situations according to chosen values. The way we think, in turn, influences the patterned reactions of the emotional brain. However, the depressed state of mind falls into a rut of negative thinking, self-criticism, and helplessness, upsetting the natural balance of the three systems of the "old brain." The threat protection system is over-stimulated, causing anxiety, anger, shame, and pessimism. The energizing and soothing systems are inhibited, resulting in fatigue, joylessness, and social isolation.

Imagine that you are attending a Beethoven symphony. The music is rich, exciting, and uplifting. The sounds of the various instruments blend together, creating harmonious beauty. If you surrender to the music, your heart soars. Captivated by the beauty, you are transported to another world and feel more alive. However, if you are in a depressed state of mind, you hear the music in a particular way. Instead of hearing the richness of all the instruments playing together, you focus all your attention on the drum. It is a drumbeat of loss, defeat, and failure. The symphony is no longer enjoyable, freeing your spirit, but painful and obnoxious. You want to cover your ears and run away.

In answer to the question opening this section, we are not all born to be depressed. Because of the emotional brain that is our biological heritage, we naturally respond to loss with sorrow. We mourn the loss and bounce back. However, if we were born into a family with a long history of mood disorders, we may inherit a brain predisposed to depression. We react to loss intensely and do not recover so easily. We get stuck in a dark mood. Studies suggest a strong genetic influence on developing both mood and addictive disorders. About 40% of our risk of depression is linked to our genes.

THE TEMPERAMENTAL STREAM: A MELANCHOLIC PERSONALITY

Our innate temperament also influences our tendencies toward both addiction and depression. Of all the personality traits, the one that stands out most for both the addicted and the depressed is a sensitivity to negative emotional states, a preoccupation with what is missing in their lives. They shoot for the stars, but feel mired in mud. They descend into the depths of their feelings, and their rational minds drown in a sea of emotion.

Carl Jung, the renowned Austrian psychologist, called the alcoholic a "frustrated mystic." Working with alcoholic patients, he observed that the craving for alcohol was equivalent to a deep spiritual thirst for wholeness. His alcoholic patients were sensitive souls who felt broken by life and undertook a frantic search to fix themselves. They sensed many competing desires, desperately sought satisfaction, and always wanted more from life. He described them as emotionally sensitive, wounded, and searching for new life. In alcohol, they found the spirit that was missing, giving them temporary relief. It gave them a sense of power and control in an emotionally overwhelming world.

Angela, a young woman sensitive to the tragic in life:

"I've always been shy and self-conscious. My family and friends complain to me that I'm too sensitive. My feelings get hurt so easily. It doesn't take much—a frown, a critical comment, even someone not saying 'hello' to me. I take it so personally and think I did something wrong. Any slight brings me to tears. No reassurance can take the pain away completely. It's tough to live in my skin. I spend lots of time in my bedroom daydreaming. I comfort myself fantasizing about a Prince Charming sweeping me away and our living happily ever after. I'm a romantic at heart. I love to read poetry and write poems when I feel most down. It helps to express all the sadness I feel inside. I can't help being so sensitive. It makes the world a cruel place for me that I need to escape. My imagination is my refuge."

Those with depression-prone temperaments are sensitive souls who feel the pain of life deeply. The Greeks called them "melancholic personalities," explaining that they had too much black bile in their bodies. Another era identified them as "tragic romantics," those who longed for a perfect love and felt deeply the disappointments of life. Psychology today suggests that those given to depressed moods possess a high level of the personality trait "neuroticism," which is a tendency to be in a negative emotional state. That sounds pejorative to me. I prefer to view this trait as "exquisite sensitivity to the tragic in life."

Those who are exquisitely sensitive tend to be shy and self-conscious. It is not that they lack social skills. They just prefer to keep their deep thoughts and feelings to themselves for protection. They feel different from other people because of their sensitivities. They may see themselves as outsiders, even outcasts. Being misunderstood, rejected, or abandoned is what they fear most. Many have felt abandoned by someone important to them and live in fear of being hurt again. They have an acute sense of loss, noticing more than others what is missing in life.

These individuals live more from their hearts than their heads. They feel deeply and can be swept away by their emotions. They engage in life emotionally and may distance themselves from their rational mind. Horace Walpole observed, "Life is a tragedy to those who feel, but a comedy to those who think." A tragic sense of unrealized dreams grips them. Their heart and imagination hold many dreams of a perfect life, mostly revolving around a loved one. Of course, storybook romances can never be fully realized. So they live with a delicious and painful sense of loss and longing. Idealists in their imaginations, they are pessimists in their emotions.

How do these sensitive souls cope with the intensity of their feelings? They may alternate between two diametrically opposed emotional reactions. They may internalize their emotions, appear timid and inhibited, and cultivate a rich imaginative life. Or they may become flooded with feeling, terrified of drowning, and release the fury of their emotional storms. Inside, they feel out of control—at the mercy of a constantly changing, threatening environment, as well as their reactions to it.

My sensitive patients often lament, "I wish I weren't so sensitive and could be like everybody else. I feel the pain so deeply."

I respond, "I know you think of your sensitivity as a curse. Perhaps it is also a blessing. You have an exquisite sensitivity that enables you to perceive things others cannot. Most people live in a narrow range of sensitivity. You sense the outliers, what is going on beyond the awareness of most people."

"How can that be a blessing?" they ask.

"It opens you to a larger world. You feel more deeply. You see more clearly so you can be compassionate with the suffering of others, with the pain they don't even acknowledge to themselves," I suggest.

Some come to appreciate and relish their uniqueness. I urge them to find some way to express their unique experience of the world. I point out how many artists are exquisitely sensitive and are tormented people who transform their suffering through their artistic work. I suggest that a creative impulse resides in their heightened perceptiveness. I encourage them to share it with others in some creative pursuit, such as writing, painting, playing music, pursuing photography, and so forth.

Unfortunately, many of the exquisitely sensitive drown in their feelings of loss. They become depressed and disengage from life. They forget the beauty and abundance in their midst. That mood may take on a life of its own, possess them, and rob them of happiness. They may also become addicted to a drug or a mood that helps them escape the world they experience as harsh and unforgiving.

THE CULTURAL STREAM: SOCIETY'S GREAT EXPECTATIONS

We live in a culture of noise, speed, and greed that fosters addiction and depression. Separated from nature's musical sounds, we are bombarded by the cacophony of modern industrial life. Car horns blare, engines roar, and people scream to be heard in crowded conditions. Everything moves at a fast pace in the name of progress. We race to reach goals, deadlines, and appointments. Billboards display what we must have to be happy. Businesses set sales goals that keep its work force stretched to the limit. More money, more toys, and more success are proclaimed as the royal roads to happiness. One author of a book on the cure for depression observed, "Human beings were never designed for the poorly nourished, sedentary, indoor, sleep-deprived, socially isolated, frenzied pace of 21st century life." (2) Addiction and depression are a symptom of and a protest against that dehumanizing culture.

Alcoholics Anonymous recognizes the impact of our driven culture on the sobriety of its members. It offers wise, counter-cultural advice as the path to both sobriety and emotional wellbeing. Using the acronym "HALT," they advocate caring for yourself. They instruct, "Don't be hungry, angry, lonely, or tired." It sounds like common sense. Neglecting these basic needs, they say, will set you up for a relapse into drinking. Interestingly, those who are depressed have problems with appetite, buried anger, social isolation, and sleep. Their basic needs go unsatisfied.

Our culture assaults us with many messages, mostly not very subtle, that fill the pool of addiction and depression. The following is a selection of those messages:

When I go to the gym, I am confronted by a sign which reads, "I can do it all in my lifetime." My exercising experience validates that message. In the gym, I am energized to push myself by upbeat music, bright lights, and two dozen televisions informing me of the latest in news, sports, and advertisements. On the surface, that sounds like a message of optimism and hope. It motivates me, like so many others, to work at having a healthy body.

What else is that message telling us subliminally? It proclaims that we have unlimited potential, that we can achieve whatever we want. We have no limits. Not even the sky is the limit. It also proclaims that we can achieve not only the perfect body we desire, defeating the aging process, but that we can do it "all." You can use your imagination and grandiose thinking to fill in the blank. Such unrealistic expectations become the seedbeds for disappointment, which underlie addictive and depressive lifestyles.

A Donald Trump biography was recently published, entitled, *Never Enough: Donald Trump and the Pursuit of Success.* The author observes, "He is a promoter, builder, performer and politician who pursues success that borders on obsession and yet, has given him almost everything he ever wanted." "Never enough" is the theme song for our culture, and Donald Trump represents one of its most accomplished crooners. The message is that we can find happiness in wanting more and more and working hard to get it. The "more" we are encouraged to pursue, of course, is money, possessions, and power. The promise is that the more we have of these commodities, the happier we will be. Happiness in life is measured by how much we have, not who we are. We find our identity in acquiring and achieving. That sounds noble, until you reflect on the reality of our mortality and realize that none of it lasts, except in the memory of others. The addicted and depressed are obsessed with their mortality and become exhausted and deflated in their pursuit of success.

"Be the best; be number one," is a mantra that closely follows the previous one. American culture takes Darwin's idea of the survival of the fittest to its extreme. The world is envisioned as a gladiatorial contest in which only a few can survive. This competitive world is divided into two groups, the winners and the losers. Even among the winners, there can be only one who is the best. All others are considered losers from this perspective. If you are not the fortunate "one," you are a failure in whatever you are pursuing. There is no cooperation, only competition and envious comparison. We do not work together. We fight each other to be the unique, singular winner. The prize is the label of being recognized as "number one" in the world, at the top of the heap. Such a competitive mentality encourages envy and despair. Addiction and depression represent an admission of defeat in the contest of life.

"All you need is love" is the refrain from a popular Beatles song. It captivates our imagination because it feeds a fantasy deeply imbedded in our culture. It is a protest against the blind, driven pursuit of success and accumulation of wealth. Instead, it proposes what Romeo and Juliet symbolize, happiness through the attainment of perfect romantic love. We are reborn through love. We find fulfillment through the love of another rather than from impersonal material possessions. It is people, not things, that bring us genuine contentment.

If you think more deeply about this promise of happiness, however, it makes another person the object of pursuit like any material object. It puts all our eggs in the one basket of relationships. Romantic love becomes the equivalent of wellbeing. Yet, remember how Shakespeare's play ends. It is a tragedy. In the end, all relationships are terminal and fail in providing a lasting happiness. Both the addicted and the depressed are exquisitely sensitive to the failures of love in their lives. Their hopes have been dashed on the rocks of abandonment and rejection.

"Look out for number one." Our narcissistic culture focuses on the one, the unique, the special. It encourages the pursuit of independence and self-reliance, the pioneering spirit that made America great. A corollary to this slogan is: "Be your own person. Take charge of your life." Such an aggressive attitude can lead to great accomplishments. It can also lead to a sense of isolation, the doing-it-on-your-own attitude of the Lone Ranger who rides off into the sunset. Unfortunately, glorification of the individual can easily slip into narcissistic self-obsession that ignores others and the common good. We then become a nation of separate, self-seeking, self-centered individuals competing with one another for limited resources. We ignore our innate need for connection. Such a sense of isolation feeds addiction and depression.

"Time is money." Henry Ford invented the assembly line to increase the efficiency of producing cars. It was a huge step forward. Wages and profits were increased. The economy grew, and cars became affordable. Efficiency became identified with progress. The most we can produce in the shortest time is the goal. Time, then, becomes our opponent. We beat it by moving faster and doing more. The result is more production, but also exhaustion. We want it all, and we want it now. Such impatience also breeds addictive and depressive tiredness and withdrawal from life.

Many streams of influence flow into the pool of depression. Their currents are strong and irresistible. The rush of these waters slowly shapes the personality, just as a river contours a landscape.

4

The Addictive Personality
The Walking Dead

"We would rather be ruined than changed.
We would rather die in our dread
Than climb the cross of the present
And let our illusions die."

—W. H. Auden

Addictive behaviors are only the tip of an iceberg that reaches deep into the psyche. As explained in the last chapter, they arise from natural, biological, temperamental, and cultural streams. Alcoholics Anonymous clearly recognizes this and teaches that addictive behavior is not the problem, only a symptom. More is hidden than meets the eye. We have to look deeper to discover the roots and causes.

The influence of ongoing addictive behavior also goes in another direction. The tip of the iceberg also moves the mass, slowly and predictably. Over time, the drinking or drug use begins to shape the personality. Once a person becomes addicted, their thinking, emotional responses, and behaviors follow a predictable pattern. These progressively engrained reactions become fixed and frozen, shaping personality and character. What results is an "addictive personality," which must be thawed and reformed for a full recovery.

Depression, like addiction, shapes the personality along well-worn paths.

We know that certain temperament traits, such as sensitivity to loss and emotional dependency, predispose individuals to develop depressive disorders. Painful life experiences and unrealistic expectations contribute to the emergence of depression in those who are genetically predisposed. However, once the depressive disorder takes hold, physical sensations and perceptions of oneself and the world shift. Ways of thinking, behaving, and reacting emotionally take a negative turn. These reactions become frozen over time, habits hard to break. You feel helpless in the grip of this dark mood.

If you are overwhelmed with sadness and sorrow, you may exhibit these personality traits:

- You are preoccupied with your painful losses and distrust any pleasure in life.

- You feel helpless and resign yourself to a life of misery.

- You see yourself as worthless and long to be rescued.

- Your feeling and thinking focus on the negative, on what is missing.

- You become childlike in your helplessness and withdrawal from life.

Let me briefly explain how being hooked on a mood can shape your personality.

PAIN PREOCCUPIED

Alcoholics seek pleasure and avoid pain, at all costs. The Steps/Traditions Book (1) observes: "Instinct run wild in themselves is the underlying cause of their destructive drinking" (p. 44). Alcoholics, in their self-centeredness, want to indulge their needs. They want immediate gratification, and without limits. They want it all, and want it now. They dive headlong into the chase.

However, the unrestrained pursuit of pleasure, chasing the "high," over time takes a demonic turn. Sooner or later they hit a wall. Drinking for the fun of it becomes drinking just to feel normal. As tolerance builds, it takes more alcohol to get the same intoxicated feeling and to dispel painful withdrawal. The physical, emotional, and spiritual damage mounts up with each drinking binge. Relationships suffer and begin to fall apart. Shame and despair eat away at their souls.

Drinking for pleasure becomes drinking to avoid intolerable pain. The pain comes not only from hangovers, but from the physical, emotional, and spiritual wreckage caused by the drinking. The Steps/Traditions Book comments on this shift: "Our lives have been largely devoted to running away from pain and problems. We fled from them as from a plague. We never wanted to deal with the fact of suffering. Escape via the bottle was our solution" (p. 74). Slowly, the solution becomes the problem. Running away from pain and problems through drinking becomes a way of life over time. But the pain and problems do not disappear when ignored. They grow in intensity and cause more suffering, becoming another excuse to drink more.

Like the alcoholic, when depressed you are preoccupied with your pain. It is always on your mind. You feel it in the tensions, aches, and discomforts of your body. Perhaps, you remember fleeting moments of pleasure. Their recollection only increases your painful sense of loss, loss of what once was but is no more. Now, you feel hopeless about ever recovering those good times. All joy is drained from your life and so is the hope of ever finding it again.

Caroline, a woman preoccupied with being abandoned:

"I attempted suicide by taking pills after my husband left me. I had no reason to live. I thought my life was over. He was the love of my life, but I really never felt secure in our ten years together. I always thought he would leave me because I'm such an unhappy person. He tried to reassure me, but the comfort would not last long. I was terrified of being abandoned, as if I'd never gotten over my father abandoning the family. What I dreaded most was my husband leaving me for another woman. I constantly questioned him whenever he came home late from work or I didn't know where he was. I scrutinized all his activities because I felt so insecure. My distrust drove him crazy. We ended up fighting all the time about it. And then my worst fears happened. He left me for another woman. Now I'm left alone with my misery."

Depressed, you feel vulnerable to loss and disappointment. You dwell on the painful losses from the past and wait in dreadful fear of something bad happening to you again. Your mind obsesses about being hurt, recalling over and over how you were wronged. Self-pity, sadness, and gloom begin to define your emotional state. Your body holds your pain. You have headaches and stomach discomfort. You feel tensions and aches throughout your body that come and go like phantoms. Your head is in a fog, unable to focus or remember. Sometimes you feel dizzy and have trouble breathing. Despair and hopelessness keep you trapped in your misery, with no confidence to escape. The black mood possesses you in your mind, body, and spirit.

Preoccupied with inescapable pain, all joy is drained from your life. You feel only emptiness. If others offer you reassurances, you reject them as lies. You do not believe you deserve any pleasures in life, so you withdraw from any activities that might be enjoyable. You feel drained of all energy and have no interest in doing anything. Your life becomes one of self-denial, a harsh asceticism. Your dark mood is like a drug that numbs you to further pain from loss and to any pleasure in life. Nothing excites you, even sex or time with a loved one. You live in a shut-down mode. Your life begins to revolve more and more around your experience of sadness and sorrow. "Misery" is your middle name.

As both addictions and depression deepen, coping with pain becomes the organizing principle of your life. Alcoholics drink more to numb the pain. Those who are depressed withdraw from life, which they view as hostile and depriving. Their illnesses consume them and make them strangers to the natural joys of life. When I asked a depressed patient what she would do if she were not so depressed, she said, "I can't even imagine. I only know myself as a sad person." Recovery comes from embracing the pain and grieving the losses.

GIVING UP ON LIFE

Alcoholics Anonymous describes alcoholism as "self-will run riot." The Steps/Traditions Book adds: "Our whole trouble had been the misuse of willpower. We had tried to bombard our problems with it" (p. 40). Alcoholics want power and control over their lives. When they run into problems, they use their mind and mood-altering drug to make the world go away. If they experience some uncomfortable feeling, like sadness, anger, or anxiety, they can make that emotion disappear in an intoxicated fog.

As the alcoholic indulges his fantasy of control with the bottle, the addiction begins to tighten its grip on his life. Believing he is exerting power over his life by drinking, alcohol becomes his master and enslaves him. Gradually, he loses his ability to choose to drink. He drinks because he needs to in order to feel normal and to avoid painful withdrawal symptoms. Even after many bitter experiences of losing control drinking, the alcoholic stubbornly insists that he can control his drinking, stopping whenever he wishes. He may even attempt to prove to himself and others that he does have control by changing what he drinks, the time when he drinks, and the amount he drinks. He may even have periods of abstinence. Nevertheless, the illness progresses relentlessly, increasing his sense of helplessness. His addiction results in a loss of control and a sense of painful resignation.

Like the addict, when you are overwhelmingly depressed, you feel helpless and trapped in your illness. The depression saps your strength. You lack the energy and will to make your life better, so you withdraw into being passive and disconnected from the flow of life. A sense of helplessness rules you.

Michael, a man resigned to helplessness:

"I hate to go out of my house. I don't have any energy or interest to go out and do anything. Occasionally, I give in to my friend's request and go out to eat with him. I push myself and end up enjoying it for a bit. Then, at some point, I become antsy and just want to go back home. My friend offers me advice on how to get out of my depression. I listen, nod my head in agreement, and then do nothing about it. I know what I do isn't normal. I look around and see other people who are happy and socializing. One thought keeps running through my mind whenever I think about making changes, 'There's nothing I can do about it.' My mother thought the same way, married to my alcoholic father. She just went along, like a martyr, and seemed to give up on life."

Another name for depression is "learned helplessness." There are many reasons why you feel so helpless. The depression saps your body of energy. You cannot sleep or eat normally, and you feel physically exhausted. Feeling agitated and restless, you cannot relax. Like a trapped animal, you may pace about, unable to sit still. Not only do you lack energy and motivation, but you cannot think clearly to organize yourself for any activity. Your foggy brain and racing thoughts interfere with your concentration and ability to remember anything. You become frustrated with yourself, imagining that you are losing your mind. When you push yourself to initiate some activity, you feel trapped in a deep hole, unable to climb out. Exhausted, you fall back in. Each futile effort to improve your life increases your sense of helplessness. So you give up in hopeless resignation.

Lacking energy, interest, or motivation, you simply sleepwalk through life. Your life slows to a crawl. As the depression darkens, you become more resigned to a life of misery with no escape. Your life loses its joy and meaning. Suicidal thoughts may come as a way of escaping the pain. You are already dead inside, so what difference would it make? You fantasize that killing yourself would be an act of asserting yourself, protesting your helplessness, taking your life into your own hands. In reality, it would be the ultimate form of giving up on yourself.

The alcoholic and the depressed withdraw into a passive lifestyle. "I can't" is their theme song. Overwhelmed with a sense of helplessness, they give up on making efforts to improve their lives. The alcoholic may imagine that he can control his life by drinking, but he soon discovers the opposite is true. The severely depressed may fantasize about escape through suicide, but such thoughts of despair only deepen their misery. Relief comes from accepting full responsibility for their lives and living according to their freely chosen values.

NEGATIVE SELF-CENTEREDNESS

You may be surprised to hear that at the heart of any addiction is self-centeredness, and not drinking or drug use. The mass below the surface of the iceberg is composed of greedy, selfish desires. The Alcoholics Anonymous Big Book (2) states: "Selfishness—self-centeredness! That, we think, is the root of our troubles" (p. 62). Drinking to get intoxicated is a selfish act. No one and nothing else matters when an alcoholic is in the midst of a binge. All cares, worries, and responsibilities are cast aside. All the pleading of family, friends, and concerned others meets deaf ears. As the addiction progresses, the alcoholic becomes more self-centered, living only for the party. Consuming alcohol becomes the organizing principle of his life, leaving little room for anyone or anything else.

The consequences of progressive alcoholic drinking inevitably lead to isolation. The Steps/Traditions Book states: "Almost without exception, alcoholics are tortured by loneliness. Even before our drinking got bad and people began cutting us off, nearly all of us suffered the feeling that we didn't quite belong" (p. 57). The self-centered, exclusive consumption of alcohol drives others away and reduces the alcoholic's social world to himself, his drinking buddies, and his bottle. The drinking leads to a lonely existence, which in turn becomes the excuse for more drinking. In the process, the alcoholic comes to hate himself, but feels powerless to stop the insane cycle.

In the throes of a dark mood, you become self-absorbed. You are not seeking pleasure for yourself, because you believe that is impossible. Perhaps the little pleasure you feel is being sedated with sleep. Mostly, your primary, or even exclusive, concern is for the relief of your pain. You see yourself as worthless. Much of your energy is invested in beating yourself up, which makes you more depressed, and not in reaching out to others. You know your merciless self-criticism is crazy, but you feel powerless to stop it. Two habits of thinking reinforce your sense of unworthiness: self-blame and guilt.

Rebecca, a woman caught up in self-blame:

"I was hospitalized after my son's divorce because I became so depressed. I felt so bad for him. His wife deserted him, and he fell apart. I felt his pain so much that I fell apart too. What made it worse for me was that I blamed myself for the divorce. Even though his father and I had a relatively happy marriage, I believed that I somehow failed him as a mother. I didn't teach him proper values and did not prepare him for marriage. When I saw problems developing in their relationship, I didn't support him enough or give him the right advice to prevent the divorce. I believed that it was all my fault. I know that's ridiculous, but I couldn't get that idea out of my mind."

David, a man preoccupied with shame and guilt:

"Growing up I attended a Bible church in which the pastor regularly gave fire-and-brimstone sermons. He talked about sin, punishment, and God's judgment. God's mercy was shoved into the background in my hearing. The sermons scared the hell out of me, but somehow gave me a vague sense of comfort. They expressed exactly what I felt about myself. As a perfectionist, I was drawn to the high ideals of the Gospel. But I always had a feeling of failure, of not being good enough. I did not follow Jesus perfectly and felt like a sinner deserving punishment."

Disposed to depression, many "shoulds" govern your life. You entertain high expectations about yourself and others. You may expect perfection, which is only an idea in your mind and is never realistic. The odds of you being perfect are zero. So you constantly feel like a failure in your all-or-none thinking. Without admitting it to yourself, you imagine that the world revolves around you and that you are somehow responsible for every bad thing that happens. You find reasons to blame yourself when others disappoint you or you do not live up to your standards perfectly. The habit of self-blame is a building block in your self-image of worthlessness and inadequacy.

Shame and guilt compound your sense of unworthiness. As you continue to fail in living up to your impossible standards, your sense of failure and guilt deepen. The more you fail, the more you fall into a trance of unworthiness. You see yourself as unworthy, defective, deficient, and flawed. Not only do you make mistakes, you view yourself, in your core identity, as a mistake. You say to yourself, "Something is dreadfully wrong with me as a person." As your depression progresses, you cling more to your story of shame, believing you deserve only punishment.

How do you find redemption? You may entertain the wish that someone will rescue you. Your hope is that you can be reborn through love. You may become dependent in your relationships, clinging to others, looking to them for reassurance that you are okay. You can become demanding in your need for love and approval to bolster your fragile self-esteem. Yet the more you hold on to others, the more desperate you feel. Your fear of being rejected and abandoned takes over. Feelings of insecurity arise, making you mistrustful of and demanding of their reassurances. You then berate yourself for being so weak and needy and isolate yourself.

Both the addicted and the depressed become self-absorbed in their illnesses. They seek relief from intolerable pain and engage in self-defeating behaviors to find it. The alcoholic withdraws into the bottle, ignores responsibilities, and alienates others. The depressed become obsessed with their unworthiness, withdraw from responsibilities, and isolate themselves. Becoming fully engaged in life and caring both for themselves and others leads to growth.

DWELLING IN DARKNESS

There is no such thing as a happy drunk. The Steps/Traditions Book presents a more accurate, sober picture of the alcoholic as one suffering emotional insecurity with the most common symptoms of "worry, anger, self-pity, and depression...guilt and self-loathing" (p. 42, 45). He feels depressed about the loss of his family, job, friends, and health due to his uncontrolled drinking. He hates himself for all the pain and sorrow he causes himself and others. Suffering follows him like his shadow.

Alcoholics suffer from distorted thinking, which takes them on a path to destruction. They are "victims of a mental obsession" (p. 22), believing that they can find happiness and escape the vicissitudes of life with alcohol. They live in a fantasy world, trying "to create reality out of bottles" (p. 100). As the addiction deepens, their lives become more and more organized around the pursuit of alcohol and "chasing the high." But, inevitably, they have collisions with reality. They crash.

Like the alcoholic, when you are depressed, you engage in one-track thinking. Your thought train moves in one direction, from and towards the negative. In your mind, you suffer one train wreck after another. Your imagined destination is oblivion. Such thinking excludes the possibility of positive outcomes, enjoyable experiences, and lasting happiness. Your pessimistic thinking, in turn, influences your moods, which proceed as inevitably as the caboose following the engine. Your mood is melancholic, dark, and heavy. It is somber, gloomy, and brooding.

Time becomes your enemy, rather than a friend that brings abundance and happiness. The past bears losses and sorrows, while the future promises danger. Two ways of thinking about the past and the future predominate: dysphoric, as opposed to euphoric, recall and worst case scenario.

Greg remembers only heartache:

"I was diagnosed recently with cancer. I'm not surprised because nothing has ever gone right in my life. Life has never given me a break. The only thing that ever gave me any satisfaction was work. And now I can't work and feel totally useless. Fate was against me from the beginning of my life. My parents never cared for us four children. They were too busy partying. Protective Services stepped in and placed us in foster care. That was jumping from the frying pan into the fire. My foster father used to beat me, until I was old enough to run away. Then, I married a woman who cheated on me, and I ended up alone. What more can go wrong?"

When you are depressed, your attention focuses on the past and all your misery. Your memory is selective, recalling only the negative events. That is dysphoric recall. You may have some pleasant memories, but the good times never lasted, only the trouble remained. Reviewing your past, you think only of your failures and what could have been. Focusing on your unhappy past makes you think of yourself as a helpless victim at the mercy of a cruel world. In a peculiar way, your identity as a victim gives you a sense of security. In the midst of your chaotic, unpredictable world, one thing is certain in your mind: You will suffer at the hands of fate.

Gertrude anticipates only catastrophe:

"I was told that your senior years are supposed to be golden years. That's a lot of bunk. Nothing could be further from the truth. Since my husband retired, we have had nothing but health problems. We had plans to travel and enjoy ourselves. I must have been naïve to think that would happen. My husband had a stroke and can hardly move around. He is moody and forgetful and seems to be getting worse

every day. I had a heart condition and surgery. I don't have any strength or interest in doing anything. I just take care of my sick husband. What does the future hold for us? Nothing good. I just see us going downhill. Death would be a relief."

Anxiety follows closely with your depressed mood. Preoccupied with so many painful losses in your life, you anticipate them continuing indefinitely. You worry about the worst happening to you. You imagine your life trend of misery continuing and even getting worse. The unknown disturbs you most. Distorting reality, you create the illusion of security with your certainty of some terrible thing happening to you in the future. Better the catastrophic known than the mysterious unknown.

For both the addicted and the depressed, negative moods and thinking provide an anchor in the swift-flowing events of life. Intolerant of change and its challenges, you find the illusion of security in your fixed thoughts and emotions. Your mood becomes a place of refuge, painful yet predictable. On the path of recovery you discover another anchor, faith in a Power greater than yourself.

STUCK IN CHILDHOOD

The Steps/Traditions Book reported a study by psychologists and doctors of a group of problem drinkers in the early years of AA. Their conclusions shocked the AA members at the time. The researchers concluded that "most of the alcoholics under investigation were still childish, emotionally sensitive, and grandiose" (p. 123).

After an initial protest, the AA membership, over time, has come to acknowledge the accuracy of the observations of those early researchers. Those in recovery have learned how much their personalities were formed to be childlike and irresponsible by their years of drinking. Driven by unreasonable fears and anxieties, they developed a false pride to compensate for their deep emotional insecurities. Like children, they became self-centered in the extreme, seeking the immediate gratification of their desires. They ignored responsibilities to family, friends, and work, seeking only to escape their pain and problems in the bottle. They avoided anything unpleasant and indulged their fantasy of creating a carefree life through drinking.

In short, the alcoholic regressed to become a child again in his obsessive pursuit of pleasure and avoidance of personal responsibility.

Caught up in your depression, you may come to realize how much you feel like a helpless child. You may even be looking for a magical, powerful parent to rescue you. You are at the mercy of your moods and feel helpless to change them. Your thinking is childlike in its simplicity. You see only the negative, not the complexity of life, which also includes the positive. You think in black-and-white terms, seeing only the black. Your mood reflects your preoccupation with darkness. It robs you of energy, motivation, and passion, making you withdraw from the challenges of living a full life. Self-absorbed, you desperately seek some relief and isolate yourself for protection.

Despite feeling like a helpless child, you know you are an adult with adult responsibilities. However, your illness makes you regress and become fixated at a less mature age. Seeing yourself in such a light makes you even more critical of yourself. You are not living up to your potential as a responsible, caring, contributing adult. You have fallen asleep on the job because you feel so dead inside. Addicted to your mood, you feel stuck in the river of life, unable to free yourself.

Despite your preoccupation with doom and gloom, there is hope. An enlightened life awaits you beyond the darkness. In fact, the pain can propel you forward on that journey back home to yourself, but it will require concerted effort. Your task will be to accept the challenge to get to know yourself in all your fullness, which includes the light with the dark. With that knowledge, you will be empowered to acknowledge where you need to grow up and take action.

PART TWO
HOMECOMING

Dennis Ortman, Ph.D.

5

The Steps
A Journey Home

"Happy the sorrowing; they shall be consoled."

—Jesus

"Everything arises and passes away.
When you see this you are above sorrow.
This is the shining way."

—Buddha

"We could have had it all," the refrain from Adele's popular song, echoes through your mind when depressed. You lament the many losses in your life. Perhaps you were born with a "chemical imbalance" that you believe keeps you from being happy. The hardship of having parents not good enough haunts you. You think about the loved ones who have come and gone in your life. All the disappointments, the failed projects, and the lost opportunities occupy you constantly. In the midst of all the changes in your life, you have a keen sense of the tragic. You fantasize about what your life could have been if fate had not been so cruel. "If only," you say to yourself. Sorrow is your constant companion.

A further disturbing thought strikes you. You are not simply a helpless victim of fate. You have been your own worst enemy. You also are responsible for your own misery. Most painfully, you ruminate about the many ways you failed personally, bringing trouble on yourself. Self-accusations and regrets possess you. You believe you deserve punishment for all your faults and failings.

Dwelling on your past losses and mistakes, you become nostalgic. You feel a painful sense of homelessness. In your sadness, you do not feel like you belong in this world. You are an outcast. You feel alienated from others, from yourself, and from life itself. There is no place you can call home. You long for some magical homecoming to peace and contentment.

Raymond, a chronically depressed man:

> *"I never saw myself as depressed. I never felt any strong emotions, either happy or sad. I was just low-keyed. I did my job every day and took care of my family. People would describe me as responsible and conscientious, a little boring, but a nice guy. My supposed serenity collapsed when my wife told me she was unhappy and wanted a divorce. I had no idea she felt so miserable and alone in our marriage. We met with a counselor to save the marriage. The counselor asked me many questions about my childhood and my feelings about my mother's drinking and the disruption it caused. I thought I had no feelings about it. I'm learning how I shut down my painful feelings to survive. It depresses me now to admit that I don't know myself. Somewhere along the line I lost myself and didn't even know it."*

The most painful loss in depression is the loss of yourself, who you really are. How do you recover, or uncover, your true self? How do you come back home to yourself?

THE TWELVE STEPS: A JOURNEY HOME

The Twelve Steps of Alcoholics Anonymous provide a guided path back to yourself. They show you a way through the darkness of your depression to enlightenment. They point the way home. AA warns that the journey of recovery is challenging and difficult, the road less travelled. "All of AA's Twelve Steps ask us to go contrary to all our natural desires…they all deflate our egos" (AA, p.55). It is a perilous path fraught with dangers and pitfalls. You are asked to venture into unknown territory, facing your fears and faults. Your demons will assault you, and you will beg for some Power greater than yourself to rescue you.

Working the Steps will stretch you beyond what you imagined and push you to give up your childlike thinking and grow up. It is a heroic journey requiring honesty, humility, and courage. You may want some quick fix. But there is no magical cure for your depression offered here. The Steps promise aid "to discover a way to live at peace with unresolved problems" (EA, p.1). Coming to peace with your black moods, you will find yourself and a renewed life.

The Steps embody the wisdom of spiritual traditions, both ancient and modern. Our great spiritual leaders undertook rigorous personal journeys to discover who they were and their missions in life. They took the road less travelled and encouraged their followers to do the same.

Moses ventured into the desert in Egypt and encountered a burning bush. He met Yahweh and was given a mission to set his people free. Moses left his shepherd's job, confronted the Pharaoh, and led the Jewish people through the desert. In the desert, they faced many trials before they entered the Promised Land.

Siddhartha Gautama, a prince in a northern Indian kingdom, left the comfort of his palace. He saw suffering he never knew existed and was resolved to find the way to relieve it. He went off into the forest to study, meditate, and starve himself, seeking an answer.

Meditating under a bodhi tree, he battled his demons and arose as the Buddha, the "enlightened one." He taught his followers to be lights unto themselves, finding a home there.

Homer's Odysseus engaged the Trojans in a ten year war. Leaving victorious, another adventure awaited him on his journey home to Ithaca, where his wife and family awaited him. His ten year voyage home across storm-tossed seas brought him face-to-face with many obstacles, both outside and within himself. Odysseus again had to prove his courage and resolve before he could reach home.

Jesus of Nazareth left home and his carpenter's job at age thirty. He wandered into the desert, like his Jewish ancestors, where he fasted, prayed, and was tempted. He emerged to be baptized by his cousin John and began a new career as a preacher and prophet of the good news. His journey was just beginning at that point. His ministry of preaching and healing took him to Jerusalem where, according to the Bible, he was crucified, rose from the dead, and returned home to His Father.

Muhammad, a successful businessman, went off regularly to the desert to pray. In a cave, he encountered an angel of God who commanded him to recite God's word to his people. He left that cave a prophet, with a mission to spread that word. That mission resulted in many battles and a return home to Mecca.

There are three common elements in all these journeys, which are the guiding lights for the Twelve Steps. They are the three "As" of recovery: awareness, acceptance, and action. Taking these steps confronts your depressive tendencies, the three "Rs:" retreating, rejecting, and reacting. Let me explain each.

AWARENESS: SEE MORE CLEARLY

Depression, like any addiction, anesthetizes you. It acts like a sedative-hypnotic that makes you sleepwalk through your life. However, it is not a peaceful sleep, but a fitful one. Your mood numbs your sensitivity to other feelings, especially joy. You only feel pain. Your depressed state of mind interferes with your ability to concentrate and think clearly. Negative thoughts of harm and helplessness fill your mind.

Some of the Steps challenge you to awaken from your slumber and get to know yourself. They invite you to stop, look, and listen to yourself and see what you discover. The word depressed is revealing. It means "pressed down." What is pressed down by your mood? It is some life force within you. The opposite of depression is not happiness, but vitality. Something alive in you is enshrouded in your mood. Your first surprising discovery will be the hidden life and power within you. You will uncover the wonder of your being.

You may think your painful dark mood is your problem. It is not. It is a symptom of some deeper problem that eludes you. Your depression may hide the more troubling pain of early life trauma or other losses you cannot bear to be conscious of. It also disguises what you cling to for happiness. The loss you dwell on reveals some attachments you cannot stand to live without. Your second surprising discovery will be the faults, false beliefs, and unrealistic expectations that underlie your mood.

A third discovery will be that there is a battle going on within you between two minds. Paying close attention to the rise and fall of thoughts, you notice the fascinating complexity of your mind. On the one hand, you have a mind of disappointment that focuses on how reality has failed to meet your needs. You observe what is missing or not living up to your expectations. It exhibits scarcity thinking. On the other hand, you think with a mind of satisfaction that recognizes what life is offering, the gifts you are receiving. Your thoughts embrace the fullness of experience and show abundance thinking.

When depressed patients come to see me, they plead, "Doctor, tell me what to do to feel better." Some see me as the expert who can rescue them magically.

"First, let's try together to understand what is going on so you can find relief," I respond. I also encourage them, to their dismay, to lean into the painful feeling, not run away from it. I assure them, "By becoming thoroughly acquainted with your mood, you will learn important things about yourself."

At the end of the session, they may ask me for some homework assignment to help relieve the pain. I encourage them, "Just pay attention to yourself. See what you notice. We'll talk about the experience in the next session."

Feeling impatient for immediate relief, some may press me for more specific advice. Acknowledging their pain, I also assure them, "As you come to understand yourself, you'll know what you need to do for yourself. You may already have some ideas about what helps at this point."

The healing power of awareness confronts your self-defeating tendency to retreat into your own world. Your depressed mood makes you self-absorbed and preoccupied with only the negative in your life. Awareness opens up your mind and heart to see yourself more accurately, as you actually are. That is true wisdom. It enables you to see the fullness of your life, with your strengths and weaknesses, your potential and liability. You come to appreciate what you have, and not just what is missing in your life. That can free you.

ACCEPTANCE: LOVE MORE DEARLY

You may become aware that your depressed mood disguises anger. Another name for depression is "anger turned inward." You may be enraged by what has been taken from you, feel powerless to do anything about it, and direct that anger against yourself. You indulge in self-criticism and self-recriminations. You judge yourself harshly. Your pessimism overflows into your view of the world. You condemn it as an unfriendly place and withdraw to protect yourself. At its root, depression is an act of violence, mostly against yourself.

Some of the Steps invite you to develop a more accepting attitude toward yourself, your life, and others. You begin by accepting your powerlessness over your moods and stop trying to manipulate yourself or your environment. You learn to embrace all your feelings with love, even the painful ones. In place of self-rejection, you acknowledge your faults, make amends, and come to forgive yourself. You also recognize how life and others have disappointed you. Life has been hard for you. The losses are real. You let go of your grievances and become a forgiving person.

When I ask my depressed patients their goals in the first session, an almost universal response is, "I want to get rid of the depression." Their urgency to escape the pain is understandable. I offer them hope for relief.

However, as we work together I explain to them, "Just getting rid of the feeling won't work in the long run. It puts you in a state of war with yourself. It's a war you can't win. Consider for a moment that your feelings are your friends. The pain is telling you that something is not working in your life. Let's try to understand what's going on." I also add,

"Healing will come by going through the pain, surviving and learning from it, not by going around it."

It takes a while for them to accept that loving themselves completely, including their "bad moods," will bring contentment more than hating a part of themselves will.

The healing power of acceptance challenges your tendency to reject yourself. Your depression breeds anger, which you direct against yourself. You hate your moods. Then you recall all your failures, hating your mistakes. Then you hate the raw deal life has given you. You end up hating yourself, suffering low self-esteem. Of course, the final act of self-rejection is suicide. Working the Steps, you come to compassion, accepting yourself as you are, not as you wish you would be. Only self-accepting love can cure you, replacing hatred and violence with kindness and forgiveness. It will open your heart.

ACTION: FOLLOW MORE NEARLY

Fighting your depression robs you of energy and motivation. You slow down and shut down. Like any addiction, it makes you withdraw from life and from your responsibilities. You only want to isolate yourself and sleep, if you are able. As the black mood takes over your life, you become more and more passive. Nothing gives you joy anymore. You stop doing what used to please you. You resign yourself to the pain and give up on life.

Some of the Steps spur you on to action to escape your passivity. They offer hope. Feeling dead inside, out of touch with your desires, you do not know what can make you feel alive. The Steps invite you to look more closely at what you value, and then to pursue it. Facing your despair, you make an act of faith, trusting in a Power greater than yourself. After making the effort to recognize your faults, you engage another in confessing them. Then you work to make amends and improve relationships. In your journey home to yourself, you are encouraged, with each step, to work the program. Unwholesome habits are broken and transformed by persistent effort.

We live in a pragmatic culture that seeks results. My depressed patients, of course, want to see measurable improvement in their lives. Viewing me as an authority, they ask, "How can I improve my life?"

"What do you want to do for yourself? What will make you feel alive?" I respond.

"I don't know what I want," they say. "Can you tell me what to do?"

"Who's the expert on you?" I ask.

"I know it should be me, but I'm not," they lament. The sad fact is that in their depression they have lost a sense of themselves, what they value, and what makes them feel alive.

However, you are not as helpless as you think. A deepening depression can gather momentum. You can let your black mood and negative thinking control your life. You feel like a puppet on a string. You only need to let go of those strings and choose to act differently. Taking positive action to improve your life, you gain strength and courage.

FAINTHEARTED HESITATION

A warning sign stands at the entrance of the path to maturity: "Not for the fainthearted." The Big Book of Emotions Anonymous underlines the need for personal responsibility and ongoing effort: "It is our responsibility to become well...If we take responsibility, we can put our past behind us and start anew, living one day at a time; but it takes conscious effort on our part" (p. 15). It also requires discipline and daily practice to uproot engrained habits of negative thinking and reacting. Working the Steps enables you to live wholeheartedly in the present moment, which is another definition of maturity. You live beyond desire and hope, not regretting the past or worrying about the future.

At some point in therapy, my patients balk at the demands of the three "As" and counter with several "buts."

"But I'm so depressed I can't concentrate or think clearly. How can therapy help?"

"Be patient with yourself. Just simply try to pay attention to yourself," I urge.

"But I feel so miserable. How can I accept my mood?"

"Have all your efforts to get rid of the feelings worked so far? Let's see how acceptance and learning from the mood works," I suggest.

"But I have so little energy or motivation. How can I push myself to action?"

"It begins with your desire to have a better life. Simply make a commitment to follow what's important to you," I recommend.

"But I'm so impatient. How long will this take?"

"As long as you need. It took you some time to get to this point. It will take time, effort, and grace to undo it," I reassure.

You walk through life under a heavy blanket when you are depressed. Your sadness has weaved that blanket with rope-like threads. You are weighed down, stuck on the path of life. No sunlight comes through. So you trudge on, disconnected from the outside world and yourself.

Recovery involves painstakingly uncovering yourself, setting your true self free. The work of recovering yourself requires unraveling the threads of the blanket through the awareness of your sensitivities, thoughts, feelings, and habitual behaviors. Total acceptance and courageous action are also demanded. These honest efforts undo the effects of all the painful losses in your life and weave a new, multi-colored garment that shows your true colors. Amazingly, that blanket is really a holy shroud. It bears the imprint of your true self.

On recovery road, you become aware of the light and dark, accept both, and let your light shine.

GUIDE TO THE GOOD LIFE

The fellowship of Alcoholics Anonymous originally used the Twelve Steps for recovery from alcoholism. Over the years, we discovered the power of the Steps at working through a variety of addictive behaviors: codependency, overeating, gambling, sex addiction, and so forth. We now realize how we can become addicted to mood states and ingrained ways of thinking and behaving. Many of us have become addicted to anxiety, depression, and even anger. No activity can escape becoming addictive if we invest too much of ourselves in it. The Steps show a path to freedom from any addiction.

Look closely at the Steps. Consider the wisdom and practical advice they contain. Upon closer examination, it is evident that they provide useful guidance, not only for those addicted, but for anyone. All of us become blue every now and then. All of us hang on too tightly to some self-defeating beliefs and behaviors. The Steps present a sure guide to the good life, based on the wisdom of the ages. An AA slogan summarizes the Steps: "Trust God; clean house; and help others."

"Trust God." The first three Steps affirm the importance of spiritual awakening as the leverage for personal transformation. All spiritual traditions teach the essential power of faith and prayer in leading a virtuous life. Anyone who has been caught up in the grip of an addiction can testify to the need for reliance on a Higher Power to set them free. Faith in the divine implies trust in the abundance and goodness of the universe and the sacredness of all life. You draw strength from that faith to transform your life.

"Clean house." The middle four Steps urge you to confront what keeps you from being your best self. In line with all the spiritual traditions, they affirm the need for a cleansing of your faults. The character defects that arise from your ego keep you from being your true self. These Steps ask several searching questions. What do you cling to and need to let go of to progress in your life? What fears hold you back? What needs to be forgiven in you? Hanging on to your faults keeps you stuck on your journey home to yourself.

"Help others." The next two Steps help you move from a self-centered life to a life in service of others. As all the spiritual traditions teach, loving others brings lasting joy. You are not as separate from others as you think. In fact, we all come from the same Source and share the same destiny. These Steps invite you to discover the unique contribution you can make to the world. They challenge you to discover your personal values and put them into practice. That is the path to peace and contentment. (The last three Steps are repetitions of the above, an invitation to practice on a daily basis.)

USING MEDICATIONS

Many people take medication for their depression. However, you may have some reservations, such as the following:

"All medications have side effects. I don't want the added problem of side effects. I don't want to be like a zombie."

"Who knows the long-term effects of taking medications? I don't want to take the chance."

"I don't want to introduce something artificial into my body. I want a natural solution so I can be myself."

"I don't want to become dependent on medications for the rest of my life. Some of them are addictive, and I don't want to become a drug addict."

"Taking medication means I can't solve my problems myself. I don't want the social stigma of being on drugs."

Several of my psychiatric colleagues, when I consulted them, told me how they approach patients with depressive disorders. They said they take an in-depth family history of the patient during the initial evaluation. If some family members suffer from mood disorders, they suspect a genetic basis for the depression. Physical symptoms of sleep and appetite problems and a lack of energy confirm the biological contribution to the depression. They then recommend that the patient take medication.

The psychiatrists begin by prescribing an antidepressant, specifically, a Selective Serotonin Reuptake Inhibitor (SSRI), such as Zoloft, Paxil, Prozac, or Lexapro. These medications can help with depression and the accompanying anxiety. However, they can have adverse side effects for some patients. The most common side effects are gastric problems, decreased libido, and weight gain. If the side effects are intolerable for the patient or the medication does not reduce the depression enough, the doctors prescribe another antidepressant. They keep trying different medications until they find some that work. There is a whole arsenal of antidepressant medications, and new ones come out regularly.

In deciding whether or not to take any medication, you need to carefully consider the benefits and risks. The psychiatrist will try to match you with the best combination of medications and the right doses to maximize the desired therapeutic effects and minimize the adverse side effects. Getting the right medication and dosage may take some trial-and-error, requiring patience on your part. Medication can help to reduce the intensity of your depressive symptoms so that you are strong enough to work on your life problems.

There is no magic pill to make your troubles disappear. Life is difficult and uncertain. Sadness will naturally arise in the face of constant change and loss. However, working the Steps can help you use your moods for your benefit, and not let them cripple you.

6

Defeated by Sorrow
Embracing the Pain

Step One: "We admitted we were powerless over our moods—
That our lives had become unmanageable."

"Midway along our road of life, I woke to find myself
standing alone in a dark wood."

—Dante Alighieri

In your depression, you find yourself standing alone on the edge of a dark wood. You feel homeless and lost. Peering into the blackness of the forest, you see a rock-strewn path. You wonder if it is the right way home. But you hesitate to enter. The unknown scares you. At least your sadness and sorrow are familiar. The path to recovery takes you into a mysterious forest with promise and unknown perils. What can move you to take the first step?

Perhaps you have suffered from depression for a long time. Pain has been your near constant companion. You have tried so many things to rid yourself of the pain: medication, therapy, self-help books, and changing your lifestyle. Yet the black mood persists. It is more stubborn than you ever imagined. The first step tells you what you must do in no uncertain terms: "You must admit defeat!" You already feel like a loser, defeated, helpless, and powerless. What more could be needed? A whole-hearted acceptance of your powerlessness over your moods, which leads you to cry out: "Please, help me!"

Your recovery begins with a step that seems simple at first glance but is surprisingly complicated. As the AA Big Book warns: "All of AA's Twelve Steps ask us to go contrary to our natural desires...they all deflate our egos" (p.55). Who wants to admit their powerlessness over any aspect of their lives? Especially if you naturally feel so helpless and hopeless in your illness, what can be gained by admitting and accepting it? "Won't that just make me more depressed?" You may ask. Let me explain the hidden wisdom of this step.

THE GREAT "WE" VERSUS THE SMALL "I"

Hooked on your dark mood, you view your life and yourself in negative terms. You see yourself as separate, different, and inferior. A sense of worthlessness preoccupies you. "I'm a nobody, and no one really cares about me," you complain. You feel unloved and unlovable, considering yourself an insignificant, small "I." An outcast, you cannot imagine yourself belonging to the great "we" of the human race.

Veronica, ashamed of her depression:

"I have no reason to be depressed. I have a loving husband and three wonderful children. We have a comfortable life, a house in the suburbs with the proverbial white picket fence. Yet I suffer terrible bouts of depression. The moods take over, and I can't do anything. It's a chore even to take a shower. I'm so ashamed that I'm depressed and don't understand it. I'm seeing a psychiatrist, but don't want anyone to know. I'm afraid they'll think I'm crazy, or just faking it."

You may feel ashamed of your condition. Out of ignorance and fear, society stigmatizes mental illness. The wound is invisible. It is so frightening because it is beyond comprehension and control, revealing the dark side of human nature. You may share society's prejudice about it, secretly thinking yourself insane. Considering your moods irrational, you wonder what is wrong with you. You view your depression as an intolerable sign of weakness, even a character defect. To avoid feeling even more abnormal and like an outcast, you hide your moods and fears. You become an actor, playing the role of a "normal person."

Jerome, fearful of being a burden to others:

"I've been depressed my whole life. At a young age I learned how to hide my feelings. I've become an expert at it. When the fears or sadness come over me, I just get more quiet and withdrawn. I never tell anybody. I don't want to dump my problems on them and become a burden to them. I don't want to ruin their day. So I just suck it up and cope the best way I can."

You find many reasons to isolate yourself. Mostly, you feel terrible about yourself and your illness. Furthermore, you feel fatigued, drained of all energy. You lack interest and motivation to do anything, especially to socialize with others. Despite everyone's encouragement to get out and do something, you withdraw within yourself.

The isolation, of course, only deepens your depression. When someone who is depressed comes to me for therapy, I know that it is the last resort. Most likely, they have tried to deny their problem or suffered repeated failures in trying to cope. They come to me defeated and humbled. I welcome them with open arms and offer hope. I acknowledge that they are taking a huge step toward recovery and rejoining the human race.

Alcoholics Anonymous began, and thrives today, as a fellowship of sufferers. They know from bitter experience that addictions are almost never conquered alone. The work of recovery is too demanding. It requires an overturning of the tendency to retreat into their own worlds and wallow in shame. In the same way, when you are possessed by a black mood, you need to challenge the urge to isolate. You need to reconnect with others, replacing the small "I" with the great "we." Talking with a partner, close friend, counselor, or minister is a good start. Joining a support group will hasten you on your journey home to yourself.

WHOLEHEARTED ACCEPTANCE

Admitting you have a problem with depression also goes against the grain. Whenever I begin therapy with a new patient, I always ask, "What made you decide to come and see me?" Invariably, the person tells me about their problem, all their failed efforts to fix it, and their sense of being defeated. I then ask them, "What would you like to accomplish by our meeting?" Again, the predictable response, "I want to feel better. I want to get rid of the depression."

"Tell me about your depression, what it feels like, when it started, and what seems to trigger the moods." I invite my patients to become observers of their shifting mood. Then I ask them, "Tell me about yourself, about your life." The question suggests a separation between themselves as a person and their mood. I explain, "It is important that you recognize that your depression does not define you as a person. It is a condition you have. We can work with it so your condition does not control you."

You may think that simply asking for help signifies an admission of the problem. It is not that simple. For example, an alcoholic may say, "I know I have a drinking problem and am probably alcoholic." He may go to therapy and meetings, but continue to relapse and not work the program. He has made a half-hearted admission. He is not fully convinced of the reality of his illness and holds himself back. Similarly, you may admit being powerless over your depression, yet not be fully engaged in recovery. You may reason to yourself, "Since I am powerless, there's nothing I can do for myself." Then, your habitual passivity takes over.

When you admit to a problem, you acknowledge and accept the total reality of your condition. That requires an accurate understanding of what you can control and what you cannot. You desperately want to get rid of your sad feelings. But is that possible? You feel powerless to improve your life. But are you really so helpless? Your life task is to learn how to live with your condition, not with a constant battle against it. I tell my patients, "You will learn that there is a hidden message in your mood. Together we will discover it."

What are the limits of your power? The boundaries of your control and influence are not always easy to define. The Serenity Prayer acknowledges the difficulty and the attitudes required: "Grant me serenity to accept what I cannot change, courage to change what I can, and wisdom to know the difference."

POWER SHORTAGE

Bill Wilson, the cofounder of Alcoholics Anonymous, observed the central problem of alcoholics, "First of all, we had to quit playing God." Anyone with an addiction, to a drug or a mood, wants complete control over their lives. They entertain the fantasy that they can be all-knowing and all-powerful, like God, and that they can manage life for their own convenience. Such a desire is the childlike wish that underlies all addictive behavior. Spoken out loud, that desire sounds ridiculous. Life is larger than anyone. What, in fact, are the limits of our control?

First of all, you cannot control many of the circumstances of your life and your own biology. You may imagine that if you were born in a healthy family with loving parents that you would be happy. You may further imagine that if you had different physical, emotional, or temperamental characteristics that you would be content. Perhaps you believe that more money, success, status, or power would bring happiness. The list of the circumstances that define your life are endless, and largely beyond your control.

Secondly, you have no control over the past. Even though you are filled with regrets and preoccupied with all the mistakes you made, what is done is done. Furthermore, all the events that shaped your life both positively and negatively cannot be changed. All of the accumulated losses that affected your mood cannot be erased. Obsessing about the past does not change it.

Thirdly, you cannot change other people. You may imagine that if other people treated you the way you want to be treated that you would be happy. You may expend much energy manipulating and coercing them to behave as you would like. Despite your efforts, they continue to do things that surprise, frustrate, and enrage you. In the end, you discover that people are free. They think, feel, and act as they want. They resent your intrusive efforts to change them.

Fourthly, you are powerless over your depressive disorder. Psychiatrists describe your condition as a "brain disease" or a "chemical imbalance." This disease profoundly affects your mood, thinking, and behavior. You were born with a brain sensitized to loss and disappointment. Perhaps you experienced an inordinate number of painful losses. You may blame yourself for having some defect of character. I remind my patients, "You did not choose your condition. You cannot control it. You cannot cure it. And your condition does not define you as a person." Indeed, it is difficult to accept that you cannot avoid much of the pain your condition causes.

Finally, you may be surprised to hear, you cannot control your thoughts and feelings. They happen automatically. These reactions arise from early emotional programming that is largely unconscious and beyond your rational control. Early life experiences shape your thinking and feeling. I remind my patients, "Your thoughts and feelings are like clouds that come and go. They come from you, but they are not you. You are the blue sky." Your consciousness is like the sky, an open space with many passing mental events.

Because of our desire to play God, to control life, we make efforts to control the uncontrollable. The results are predictable. We experience failure.

FATED TO FAIL

When you feel the pain of depression, you naturally seek relief. You may take medications, participate in therapy, and try to change your lifestyle. You may challenge your negative thinking, making efforts to be more positive. You may even attempt less conventional treatments, like shock therapy, acupuncture, or transcranial magnetic stimulation. These treatments may provide some relief, but cannot address the roots of your sorrows. A different approach is needed.

You may develop a lifestyle organized around coping with your insecurity and not fully realize it. Engaging in these behaviors, which prove to be self-defeating, only increases your depression.

James, terrified of being abandoned:

"I find it hard to say 'no' when anyone asks me to do something. I don't even stop to think whether or not I really want to do it. I just say 'yes.' Afterwards, I often regret that I agreed. I end up doing so many things I really don't want to do. Then, I become resentful, mostly mad at myself for going along. I'm such a weakling. I've analyzed why I do this over and over. I think I'm afraid the person will not like me if I refuse to do what they ask. That's ridiculous, but I keep doing it anyway."

Raymond, a man easily overwhelmed:

"I hate that I'm such an anxious person. I get easily overwhelmed by things, so I hold myself back. I stay home most of the time because I'm afraid to mix with people. I'm afraid of making a mistake and embarrassing myself. On my job, I never push myself. I know I have talents. I just sort of hide out at my desk, doing what is expected of me, and not socializing with my coworkers. It depresses me to think about how I'm wasting my life. But I can't change."

Samantha, a control freak:

"I'm terrified of any kind of change. Everything I do is planned, sometimes to the smallest detail. I have a routine for every day of the week, and I expect my husband and children to follow that program. When they don't, I fly into a rage. Afterwards, I feel terrible about it and apologize profusely. I hate myself for acting that way, but I can't help it."

"The best laid schemes of mice and men…" Many of your strategies to manage your life end in failure. With the best of intentions, you try to cope with your moods and fears. Like James, you may become an accommodating person. Like Raymond, you may withdraw from uncomfortable activities. Like Samantha, you may create a protective wall of rules, routines, and rituals, which you aggressively protect. Life is bigger than you. Your efforts to manage it defeat you, making you feel more depressed.

What, then, do you have power over in your life? What can you manage effectively? Defeat shocks you. It jolts you to look deeply within yourself to discover where your true freedom and power lie. Where are you free? You can choose your attitude toward your thoughts, feelings and what happens to you. And then, you are able to choose how to act accordingly. Indeed, that is good news!

PAIN, THE TEACHER

The first challenge of defeat is to change your attitude toward pain. Our natural instinct is to seek pleasure and avoid pain, at nearly all costs. The first step, like all the Steps, asks you to act contrary to your natural desires. You want to avoid and rid yourself of the discomfort your depression causes you.

Much to their surprise, I invite my patients, "Lean into your pain. Don't avoid it. Learn the message of your mood." Such an approach presents an alternative path to freedom.

What would your life be like if you never felt pain?

Initially, you might think it would be heaven on earth, a dream realized. Your life would proceed pleasantly without the distraction of pain—until you injured yourself. You might not even notice you hurt yourself because you feel no pain to alert you. You do not seek treatment. The cut may become infected, and eventually cost you a limb, or worse, your life. You may become afflicted with an infinite variety of illnesses and not even know it. Without treatment, a simple sickness could become complex, damaging vital organs, and, again, costing you your life. We ignore the signs at our own peril.

Physical pain, as much as we hate it, serves a survival purpose. It alerts us to harm that requires attention. Pain grabs our attention and launches us on an exploratory search to find its cause. When we understand clearly the cause, we can move towards the proper remedy.

Emotional pain serves a similar survival purpose, to protect our psychological wellbeing. When you feel anxious, depressed, or angry, it is a warning sign that something is out of balance in your life. Of course, you hate the discomfort of these feelings and wish they would magically disappear. But these emotional reactions are symptoms of some deeper problem that is calling out for attention. Neglecting to address that deeper problem can put your long-term happiness at risk. Taking the pain seriously and exploring the causes can lead to growth.

Imagine that your hand is frostbitten. Your hand is numb. You feel no pain. However, as your hand begins to thaw, you feel excruciating pain. You think your condition is worsening, but actually, you are in the process of healing. In the same way, when you feel your sorrow fully, you are beginning to heal.

Sadness and sorrow reflect your sensitivity to loss. These reactions alert you that something you value is missing. What would life be like if you never felt sadness? Perhaps you imagine a life of perfect peace and tranquility. Think again. You could only avoid sadness if you never felt an emotional connection to someone or valued something. If you never felt sorrow, you would be emotionally dead. You could not experience joy in life. Sadness and sorrow soften your heart so you can feel compassion. These natural reactions also motivate you to find out what is missing and do something about it. Tears can be a gift.

WATCH THE FLOW

The second challenge of defeat is to change your relationship with your thoughts, feelings, and physical sensations, rather than make a futile and artificial effort to change them. You cannot effectively manipulate yourself into thinking, feeling, and reacting differently. Your thoughts, feelings, and sensations emerge from a stream of consciousness with deep unconscious roots. They come and go in an endless stream. Nevertheless, you are always free to decide how much weight you give them and how to act on them. There is no irresistible thought or impulse. You only think that. And you can decide not to act on an urgent thought or feeling.

I invite my patients, "Imagine your stream of consciousness as a waterfall. You can respond in a few different ways to the flow. You can try to stop it, jump into the river, or watch it." Let me explain.

First, you can try to stop the flow, by ignoring it or distracting yourself with other thoughts and activities. But the pressure builds, and the unwanted thoughts, feelings, and impulses erupt with a vengeance. Or they seep through in indirect ways, influencing your behavior without your awareness. What you resist persists.

The second approach is to jump into the stream of consciousness, give up any effort to manage the flow, and risk drowning. In the midst of a panic attack or black mood, you feel powerless to resist the urgent rush of threatening thoughts and feelings and are overwhelmed. You get carried away against your will.

The third approach, the only really effective one, is to become an observer of the flow of your thoughts, feelings, and physical sensations. It is like standing back and watching a waterfall, without trying to dam it or jump in. With practice, you can learn to become an astute observer of yourself and your ongoing flow of thoughts, feelings, and sensations. Taking in the information, you learn from the flow. You gain valuable information so you can decide how to act in your best interest. The more you practice observing, the more you develop habit strength to transform your life.

PAY ATTENTION TO YOUR BODY

Your body holds the pain of a lifetime of enduring losses, from infancy to the present. No wonder you have so many aches and pains when you are depressed. Your body constricts in reaction to the losses. Particular areas of your body may be more vulnerable than others to the stress of life. Your heart is heavy under the weight of the losses. You may have headaches, backaches, stomachaches, or joint pain. The physical distress keeps you from eating and sleeping normally. You may experience fatigue, or a lack of sexual drive or vitality from a lifetime of coping with loss. Your body does not lie. Your mind may be fooled. Your emotions may play tricks on you. But, again, your body knows.

A woman came to me for therapy because she had stomach pains and thought her cancer had returned. Her oncologist had given her a clean bill of health, but she still obsessed about the cancer. I asked her, "Have you ever experienced that kind of pain before?"

She responded, "Yes, while growing up. My parents fought constantly, and I had stomach aches."

"What might be bothering you now? What is hard for you to digest?"

She thought for a moment and said, "Well, my son is getting married next month. But I'm happy for him." She paused and then added, "I don't get along with the new in-laws. There have been some disagreements preparing for the wedding."

Your body cries out for attention. It alerts you to problems before even your mind recognizes them.

Medical doctors, psychiatrists, and psychologists, whether they advocate or oppose medication, encourage caring for the body when depressed (1). For example, these doctors advise:

- Regular physical exercise.

- Good sleep.

- Hygiene.

- Proper diet with supplements, especially omega-3 fatty acids.

- Sunlight exposure.

- Social support, especially staying connected with close family and friends.

- Engaging activities, a creative outlet, and mindful relaxation.

"A healthy mind in a healthy body," timeless wisdom proclaims. Our minds and bodies are not as separate as we imagine. By caring for your physical needs, you improve your mental health.

PARADOX OF WEAKNESS AND STRENGTH

When depressed, you are preoccupied with being helpless, weak, defeated, and trapped. Naturally, you want to escape. Your mind runs on a single track towards the negative. Its way stations are bad fortune, misery, disappointment, and pessimism. You know that those persistent dark thoughts keep you down. How can you derail that thought train?

Alcoholics Anonymous offers many slogans for recovery that provoke an alternative consciousness and way of living. They affirm that you can change your life by changing your thinking. These slogans express a hidden wisdom in a surprising way that contradicts your ordinary one-track thinking. They are called paradoxes, which means "a union of opposites." What you think cannot go together is really intimately related if you look more deeply. Paradoxes invite you to see wholeness, rather than contradictions, in the world around you. They challenge your usual either-or thinking to see more inclusively, in both-and terms.

Step one suggests the paradox: "From weakness comes strength." Within weakness is found the seed of strength, just as strength foreshadows weakness. Weakness and strength are really two sides of the same coin. You do not have to reject your moods or your feelings of weakness. Instead, accepting your powerlessness over your moods opens the door to new life. Pain propels you to undertake a personal journey in search of healing and growth. The suffering, if accepted, opens your heart to personal responsibility and compassion for yourself and others.

The book of Chinese wisdom, *Tao Te Ching***, expresses clearly this truth:**

> Failure is an opportunity.
> If you blame someone else,
> there is no end to the blame.
>
>
> Therefore, the Master
> fulfills her own obligations

and corrects her own mistakes.
She does what she needs to do
and demands nothing of others (79).

In the midst of your failure and sense of powerlessness in managing your moods, you have a choice. You can give up in despair and blame others, your circumstances, or fate for your misery. You can choose to remain a victim of your moods. Or you can shift the focus to yourself and take responsibility for your own life. You can stop blaming, demanding, and expecting to be rescued. You can look seriously at your own life, over which you have power, and make decisions based on your deepest desires and true values. Embracing your weakness, you find the strength to grow up.

EXERCISE: BODY SCAN

Your depressed mind often takes possession of you, and you become lost in your thoughts. You dwell on the past and all your misfortunes. You may feel sorry for yourself and seek sympathy from others. But it only makes you more miserable. In the process, you remain stuck in the past.

How can you escape the fixed negative thinking of your depressed mind? By coming home to your body and listening to its wisdom. Without knowing it, when you become depressed you disengage from your body and your experience of the present moment. By focusing your attention on your body, you anchor yourself in the present moment and let go of your thoughts about past troubles. That opens you to the future.

The body scan is a traditional Eastern practice that cultivates awareness of the body (2). The procedure is simple:

Lie down on your back in a comfortable position. Find a quiet place where you will not be disturbed. Close your eyes to avoid any distractions. Relax and feel the solidness of the floor supporting your body.

Focus on the rising and falling of your breath. Your breath signifies life and your connection with the world. Breath is also spirit. Feel yourself relaxing as you pay attention to the rhythm of your breathing. As thoughts arise, do not fight them. Simply acknowledge them and let them pass.

Shift your attention to various parts of your body, beginning with the top of your head. Slowly move your awareness through your body to the tips of your toes. Pause to notice any sensations of tension or pain. Note the quality and intensity of the discomfort. Your body, more than your mind, holds emotional pain going all the way back to childhood.

Imagine breathing into the various parts of your body as you scan it with the light of your awareness. Feel the lightness of your breath infiltrating and lifting any areas of tightness and heaviness. Stop at areas where you feel pressure and consciously breathe in the tension. Then breathe out calmness and peace.

Finally, be aware of the sense of your body as a whole. Feel yourself united and at peace with your body. Be totally relaxed.

Do this exercise in an unhurried manner for at least fifteen minutes. Afterwards, arise slowly to resume your day. Carry with you the freeing experience of being completely in your body and not in your mind. At various times of the day, pause for a moment to pay attention to your body, briefly scanning for any sensations.

"The journey of a thousand miles begins with one step," says Lao-tzu (64). Pain and powerlessness push you to take that first step. You suspect recovery will be arduous and filled with obstacles. The final destination is unknown, shrouded in mystery. The next step of hope will give you the courage to carry on.

Abundance
Coming to Faith

Step two: "We came to believe that a Power greater than ourselves could restore us to sanity."

"No problem can be solved by the same consciousness that caused the problem in the first place."

—Albert Einstein

Your pain and sense of powerlessness have moved you to take the first step into the dark forest. The smothering blackness terrifies you. Suddenly, you see a glimmer of light from a distance. You wonder where it is coming from. It appears as a flickering flame, a candle in the wind, not the bright spotlight you hoped for to dispel the darkness. The light is enough to reveal a winding, rock-strewn path, overshadowed by hanging tree branches. The light gives you enough courage to begin the journey.

The second step inspires hope for your recovery. Overwhelmed by your depressed mood, you feel lost in a valley of despair. You lack the energy and motivation to climb out on your own. This step encourages you to open your mind and heart to believe in a Higher Power that promises an abundant life. It addresses several questions about finding that Power:

- How? Through coming to believe.

- Where? Beyond/within/among/around you.

- Why? To restore you to sanity.

- When? In the present moment.

• Who and what? These questions will be addressed in step three.

TODAY'S CRISIS OF FAITH

The step from admitting your powerlessness to believing in a Higher Power is a daunting one. Perhaps your depression drained your soul of faith and hope. Perhaps also you feel a sense of disillusionment with religion. You are not alone.

Recent polls document the severity of the crisis of faith and religion today (1). Almost a fifth (16 to 20 percent) of the population declare themselves unaffiliated with any church or having no religion. Many are either agnostics or atheists, and some say they are "spiritual." The young are especially skeptical. Between 25 and 30 percent of adults under age thirty claim no religious affiliation. America's third largest religious group currently is composed of those who profess no faith. Even those who belong to a church do not practice regularly. Only about 20 percent attend weekly services.

Religious institutions have taken a hit in the past two decades. Several events have disillusioned many Americans (2). The terrorist attacks of September 11, 2001, awakened the world to the reality of religious fanaticism. Politicians blamed Islam, and preachers blamed American infidelity for the attacks. Religion in general looked bad. The clergy sex abuse scandal in the Catholic Church shocked both believers and nonbelievers. What outraged most was how the bishops covered up the abuse to protect the image of the Church, at the expense of innocent children. The Protestant infighting over gay priests and bishops revealed a mean-spiritedness that contradicted the Gospel. Christianity began to appear to be a religion for the judgmental, bigoted, and socially insensitive. Finally, the conservative agenda of the religious Right, which supported George W. Bush, alienated an entire generation of young people. Their views on women, same-sex marriages, the environment, and global poverty did not align with Gospel values, as interpreted by the liberal youth. These events provoked a mass exodus from the churches.

Recent surveys report that only about 20 percent of Americans say they have a "great deal" of confidence in organized religion. Churches today do not represent the open-minded, compassionate spirit of their founders. Many young people have intensely negative views of Christianity, accusing its members of being anti-homosexual, judgmental, hypocritical, and out of touch with reality.

The spirit of our age also challenges faith. Our culture proclaims, "Only seeing is believing." Only what can be perceived by the senses is considered real. If you cannot observe and measure it, it is thought a figment of your imagination. The sensory, empirical, material world is all there is. Happiness can be found only by immersing yourself in that world and pursuing its pleasures. This view of the world has been called "flatland." You live on the surface of life, ignoring both its depths and heights. Talk about God, the soul, and the afterlife sounds like nonsense because it cannot be verified by proof.

A SLEEPING SPIRIT

Your depression can be a gateway to a spiritual awakening. As an AA saying observes, "Religion is for people who are afraid they'll go to hell. Spirituality is for people who have been there." However, if your dark mood takes over your life, you may resist opening your heart to faith.

Erica, disheartened by despair:

"I've been depressed my whole life. It seems I was born to be unhappy. My parents took me to counselors and psychiatrists. They were devout Catholics and took me to church every Sunday. They tried to encourage me in my sadness. 'Just have faith in God,' they said. When I think about God I become angry. 'How could a good God create me to be so miserable?' If there is a God, He is cruel, not loving. I really don't believe in God or heaven. I do believe in hell, though. I'm living there now."

George, obsessed with control:

"My life changed dramatically twenty years ago when I injured my back in an auto accident. Since then I've lived with chronic pain. Some days it's barely tolerable. I refuse to take pain medication because I never want to lose control. I'm terrified of becoming addicted. So I just cope the best I can. To be honest, I think about the pain all the time, how much I hate it. I know I can't control it, but I'm obsessed with how miserable it makes me and with getting rid of it. My obsessing about it only makes it worse, but I can't help myself."

HOW TO BELIEVE IN THE POWER

Taking a leap of faith may terrify you. It defies your natural instincts for control, certainty, and clarity. Let me present a view of faith that may respond to some of your objections. Believing concerns:

- A journey, not a destination.
- The unknown, not the known.
- Letting go, not hanging on.
- The heart, not the head.
- Opening, not closing.
- A gift, not a reward.
- Here and now, not then and there.
- A lifestyle, not a belief system.

1) A JOURNEY, NOT A DESTINATION.

Coming to believe is a lifelong journey that is never complete. It begins with the desire to believe and may take many twists and turns before you arrive at a decision of faith. You may find yourself hesitant to take that leap of faith. As a reasonable, even scientific-minded person, you do not want to sacrifice your intellectual integrity, accepting what you cannot understand. You will not tolerate blind obedience. Talk about God may not make sense to you, and you do not see any connection between faith and your emotional problems. Even after you make the decision, the journey continues. Unexpected life events challenge your faith, creating doubt and the need to renew the exploration.

Whatever your reservations, you do not need to rush to belief until you are ready. All that is required is an open mind and heart and a willingness to search for a deeper truth in life.

2) THE UNKNOWN, NOT THE KNOWN.

As a depressed person, you hate change. Change creates painful loss and an unknown future. To give you a sense of security, you dwell on your past, on what could have been. It feels less threatening than the future, which is unknown, uncertain, and unpredictable. You create in your mind a predictable future by imagining that the worst case scenario will always happen. The future will simply repeat your unfortunate past. You choose to live on the surface of life with your conscious pessimism.

Faith invites you to look deeper, beneath the surface of everyday life. Believing draws you into the darkness of the unknown, which is beyond your understanding and control but from which all knowing arises. It is a journey to the Center and Source of life, which is shrouded in mystery. Despite your anxiety about the unknown and your desire for solid ground, you know that you cannot completely reduce the mystery of life into what you can manageably know. You sense that being comfortable with the unknown, the unpredictable, and the unfamiliar is essential for you to be free to live a full life.

3) LETTING GO, NOT HANGING ON

You cannot make faith happen. You cannot force yourself or anyone else to believe. Instead, you have to open your mind and heart to the mystery of life, to the completely new and unexpected revealing itself. That requires letting go of many of your assumptions about life.

If you are depressed, the change you resist most is changing your mind. You live in the past, remembering all your hurts and regrets. You feel powerless to stop your obsessing, even though you recognize its harmfulness. You firmly believe you are worthless and powerless and that fate is against you. For the sake of security, you believe you need to hang on tightly to these beliefs. A variation of Murphy's Law becomes your credo, "If anything can go wrong, it will—because it always has."

To make room for faith, you have to surrender these fixed ideas and open yourself to the possibility of surprise and wonder.

4) THE HEART, NOT THE HEAD

Faith does not contradict reason, but you cannot reason yourself to believe. The mystery of faith goes beyond the thinking mind and engages you at a deeper level. You believe with your whole person, your mind, heart, and soul. It requires a wholehearted trust, a heart-consciousness that engages you at the core of your being.

As much as you think your sorrowful emotions dominate you, the truth is your distorted thinking controls you. You are a prisoner of your pessimistic thinking. You are lost in your thoughts about terrible things happening. Preoccupied with these negative ideas, you become disengaged from yourself. Your thinking mind analyzes, judges, manipulates, and distances you from yourself and others. Your chattering thoughts distract you from the subtle whisperings of your heart. At some level, you may sense that you are addicted to your negative way of thinking and feel powerless to change it.

You long to live from your heart, not your head, knowing that is the path to a richer life.

5) OPENING, NOT CLOSING

Faith involves a journey to a sunlit mountaintop where you can see forever. It is a new state of consciousness open to the fullness of life, where you see that everything belongs. Nothing is excluded. Even what you fear and despise can be incorporated into your path to a wholesome life.

Living in the dark pit of your depression, you withdraw from the world to protect yourself. Your mind is imprisoned in negativity. Past hurts preoccupy you. Shutting down your feelings, you close yourself off from experiencing joy in life. You hibernate in that black hole. Your mood sucks all the life out of you. Disengaging from your usual activities and from socializing, your world shrinks. The leap of faith can seem overwhelmingly frightening because it means giving up the past you cling to so desperately.

Faith beckons you to climb out of the hole and look at life differently. It invites you to embrace your losses, opening your mind and heart to the new life that will emerge.

6) A GIFT, NOT A REWARD

Coming to faith is coming to enlightenment. It is a gift which cannot be earned. You can prepare the ground, making your heart ready to believe, by slowly accepting the inevitable suffering that life brings. But you cannot make faith blossom. That power eludes you, which is a cause for humility.

In the grip of gloom, you feel helpless and hopeless. You lack the energy and motivation to work for faith. However, your pain and sense of powerlessness are the soil needed for faith to grow. Feeling so desperate and broken awakens your longing for a Power greater than yourself to bring relief. As Leonard Cohen wrote, "There is a crack in everything. That's how the light gets in."

7) HERE AND NOW, NOT THEN AND THERE

Many despise religion because it takes them out of the world. It promises heavenly rewards in the afterlife. The mission of believers, then, is to endure the trials and tribulations of the present life with the hope of a better life later.

That is a distortion of authentic faith. Believing involves being fully engaged in the present moment, which reveals the divine presence. It means taking this life seriously, making this world a better place as the path to happiness. The eternal is found in the everyday. Here. Now.

Your moods prevent you from living fully in the present moment. Time and change are your enemies. You ruminate about past hurts, preoccupied with endings. You worry about the unknown future, which threatens more harm. So you feel stuck in time. You cling to the familiar endings and dread new beginnings.

The distress of regret and worry may awaken a longing in you to seek refuge in the present moment, a necessary condition for faith.

8) A LIFESTYLE, NOT A BELIEF SYSTEM

Believing is not simply a matter of professing a creed, of saying, "I believe in God." Many of you reject religion because so many professed believers do not practice what they preach. They talk about the God of love, but live in hateful ways. They preach the golden rule, but live self-centered lives. Common sense says that you get a more accurate reading of what someone believes by watching the feet, not the lips.

Authentic faith is more about actions than words. It is embracing a way of life guided by a belief in the Ultimate Source of Love. The Dalai Lama expressed this beautifully when he said, "My religion is kindness." Genuine faith overflows in a life of virtue, which is its true mark. Coming to faith will require you to give up your preoccupation with being wounded, which interferes with freely loving others.

WHERE'S THE POWER?

At the heart of depression is resistance to change. Change involves inevitable loss, death. You have difficulty imagining a new life, a new beginning, emerging from the loss. You feel helpless and hopeless in the throes of change. Where do you find the Power to negotiate the many transitions in life? What can give you hope? T.S. Elliot suggests looking "at the still point of the turning world…except for the point, the still point, there would be no dance, and there is only the dance" (3). Where is the still point, the Source from which the Power radiates to turn the world?

Darrell, lost and seeking:

> *"Since being depressed I lost faith in God. Not just in God, but in life. I had little reason to live. I was raised Catholic, but hadn't been to church in years. My cousin, who knew I was depressed and lost, said, 'Why don't you come with me to this great church I discovered.' After some coaxing, I went with her to a service. It wasn't like anything I'd seen before in the Catholic Church. The place was alive and exciting. People were friendly and welcoming. The music was upbeat, and the people actually sang. The preacher gave an inspiring sermon, and I wanted to listen. I've been going for several months now. There's a glimmer of hope in my life."*

As a psychologist, and not a preacher, I do not initiate discussions about faith with my patients. However, if they bring up the issue, I explore it with them. We talk about their experience of God, and I ask them, "What is your ultimate concern in life? Where do you look to find the Power for your life?" You can look in four directions:

- Beyond—towards God, the Supreme Being.
- Around—towards the Life Force of nature.
- Among—towards divine Love.
- Within—towards the indwelling Spirit.

If you are a religious person, you may look beyond yourself and put your faith in God, the Supreme Being. Attending church, praying, and performing devotional practices may give you a sense of God's loving presence in your life. You see God as a loving Father (or

Mother) who nurtures, guides, and protects you. You may read the Bible and hear God's message of love and forgiveness. As you worship, you lift up your mind and heart and feel connected to all God's people. Praying, you find comfort in your sorrows.

When you walk on the beach, hike through the mountains, or stroll through the woods, what do you experience? Simply being outdoors, sitting in your garden and listening to the birds, what do you feel? Stop your chattering mind with all its regrets and worries. Pay attention with all your senses. The experience may awaken you to a Power and glory beyond, around, and within you. You marvel at the abundance of life and sense the Life Force that sustains it. Nature uplifts and heals.

"Love makes the world go 'round," the song refrain goes. It is the energy for connection. When you are in love, you experience an energy between you and your partner that makes you feel alive. Through love, you are reborn. Love also holds communities together. Trials especially become occasions for love to show its power. The fellowship of Alcoholics Anonymous acknowledges the critical importance of coming together as a group. Many members view the group as the Power greater than themselves. They rely on the group for support and sacrifice themselves to maintain it. It is no wonder that God is defined as Love in the Bible. The one God is a community of persons, Father, Son, and Holy Spirit, bonded by love.

You may also look within yourself, intuiting a hidden power. The Spirit of God dwells within you. You see signs of it in your abilities to reason, create, make free choices, and love. These are divine qualities that you possess. These qualities separate you from the animal and plant worlds and, at the same time, lead you to care for the universe. Observing yourself closely, you perceive your own dignity as a child of God. You are filled by the abundance of God's love.

That power within yourself is your true self, which is hidden by the dark clouds of depression. Yet you do not own or create that power within. There is a paradox of power: it is yours, but not yours. It comes from a Source beyond you, yet within you. It is a divine, sacred presence that you may call God. You are "made in the image and likeness of God." His life dwells within you. You are one with God, yet not God. In coming to know yourself, you discover the Divine, the Ultimate Reality, at the heart of your being. In searching for God, you come to know yourself at the deepest level. As the great Saint Teresa of Avila said, "You find God in yourself and yourself in God."

WHY THE POWER?

What purpose does faith serve for your life now? This step provides the answer, to restore your sanity.

How can you restore your sanity? The key word is "restore." You seek to recover something that is lost, to find your original sanity, which is hidden behind the cloud of your anguish. That may seem surprising to you. You may have always felt crazy with your moods. In fact, you may have told yourself, "My middle name is depression." That is who you are. Perhaps you have never known a time when you were not sad.

Beneath your sorrowful façade lives a sane person. Your true nature is wholeness, health, clarity, and peace, but it has been clouded over by your depressed state. Your depressed mind is like a glass filled with muddy water. When the glass is shaken by loss, the silt from the bottom fills the whole glass. No light can shine through the muddy water. As long as you are agitated, the dirty water remains stirred up and opaque. When you learn to calm yourself, the sediment settles to the bottom of the glass. The water, then, becomes clear, and light can shine through. The natural state of your mind is clean, fresh water through which the bright light of truth radiates.

Patients come to me in distress, seeking change. They are surprised when I tell them my view of therapy. I explain, "Therapy is not a self-improvement project about creating a better version of yourself. Instead, it is about allowing yourself simply to be yourself, and removing any obstacles to being your true self."

Recovery involves letting the muddy waters of your agitated emotions settle. The calming permits natural wisdom, strength, and compassion to shine forth. It releases the power of your true self.

Insanity has been described as thinking and doing the same thing over and over again while expecting a different result. It is a contradiction between thoughts and actions and your expected outcomes. Your mind takes the lead in this merry-go-round. As the great psychologist, the Buddha, stated, "All that we are is the result of what we have thought: we are formed and molded by our thoughts." There is a natural sequence. Your thoughts mold your actions, and your expectations shape your mood.

Stuck in your depressed mood, filled with despair, you may think you've lost your faith. Actually, your faith is strong. It is only distorted, muddying the waters of your life. You've developed a belief system that is out of touch with reality. Without realizing it, you've developed a rigid set of dogmas about yourself and life that you hold with unshakeable faith.

Pay close attention to the silent assumptions you hold about your life. Notice what you believe you absolutely need to be happy. Without it, you think you will be miserable. The following are some examples. You may say to yourself, "To be happy, I believe I need..."

- "to have a close, loving relationship; without being loved, I cannot survive."

- "to be successful at everything I do; if I'm not, I'm worthless."

- "to be liked by everybody, to have their approval; their criticism will destroy me."

- "to have complete control over my life, or I'll be helpless and lost."

- "to have more money, possessions, and fame, or I'll be dissatisfied."

- "to be perfect, or I'm a failure."

- "to have a different past, or I'll continue to be miserable."

Notice what you feel is lacking in your life and examine your beliefs about it. You may have come to believe that you are worthless and helpless and that the world is hostile and depriving. Observe also the impact of your unrealized expectations on your mood. Make it a habit to notice your shifting beliefs.

PARADOX OF FAITH AND DOUBT

Paradoxes invite you to search your soul for their deeper meaning, as they resonate in your heart, not your logical head. You cannot fully grasp their meaning, but can sense their truthfulness at a deep level you cannot yet understand. They suggest that you embrace what confuses and distresses you to explore deeper meaning. Their message is clear: all is connected, everything belongs, and all is one. Beneath the brokenness, there is an underlying wholeness. At a deeper level, everything radiates from a Center, an abundant Source.

Step two suggests the paradox: "Through doubt we come to faith." Doubt creates confusion and insecurity for you. Your natural instinct is to crave control, certainty, and clarity. Without this, you feel lost and depressed. To compensate, you develop fixed ideas and beliefs about yourself and the world to remove any doubts. You are absolutely certain you are worthless and helpless and that the world is a terrible place. No one can convince you otherwise. These frozen thoughts are like ice, interfering with the natural, free flow of your thinking.

The darkness of doubt creates a longing for warm sunlight to thaw your fixed ideas and beliefs. Allowing yourself to doubt enables you to confront the emptiness of your ideas. It invites you to trust more in your immediate experience and to explore more deeply the mystery of life. Doubt can be creative because it opens your mind and heart to that mystery. Life is infinitely more than your fixed ideas about it. Entering the darkness of doubt prepares you for the leap of faith, through a deeper darkness, into the light. As T.S. Elliot wrote, "I said to my soul, be still, and let the dark come upon you, which shall be the darkness of God" (4).

WHEN OF POWER: NOW—FOLLOW YOUR BREATH EXERCISE

Your depressed mind jumps around with thoughts of loss and catastrophe. An ancient eastern practice to help calm the mind is called, "Samadhi," which means, "abiding in peace" (5). It is a practice that can help you concentrate, calm yourself, and experience peace. In the process, you experience your own inner power by consciously focusing your attention, which you can control with practice. You deliberately stand back and observe the passing thoughts, feelings, and sensations without being caught up in the drama.

The practice involves the discipline of focusing your attention on one thing, your breath. You exercise your "attention muscle," which, like all muscles, strengthens with use. Why focus on the breath? The breath represents life, freedom, and connection in the present moment. Breathing oxygen, you are alive; when you stop breathing, you die. Your breathing keeps you in the present moment. As a bodily function and immediate experience, you cannot drift into the past or the future, as your depressed mind tends to do with its wayward thoughts.

The procedure for this practice is simple:

1) Find a quiet place, away from as many distractions as possible. Sit in a relaxed position with your back erect and your head straight. You may sit in a chair with your feet firmly planted on the ground and hands on your lap, palms facing upward in a position of receiving a gift. You may prefer to sit in the traditional lotus position, with your legs crossed, but that is not necessary. Whatever your preferred posture, feel as though you are grounded. Keep your eyes closed to avoid distractions. Begin with the intention to pay full attention only to your breath.

2) Next, breathe deeply from your abdomen. It is important to breathe deeply, from the center of your body, and not in a shallow manner as you do when anxious and depressed. Breathe regularly and sense the fresh air filling all parts of your body. Scan your body and notice the areas of tension. Consciously send your breath to those areas and feel the warmth of your breath bring relaxation. Let the frozen tension melt away. Breathe slowly and regularly, not quickly and unsteadily. Find comfort in the regularity of your slow, deep breathing.

3) Now focus all your attention on the rising and falling of your breath. You may begin by counting your breaths and noticing the gap between inhaling and exhaling. Follow the sensation of your breathing and its movement through your body, from your stomach, through your chest and windpipe, and out your nose. Become body-conscious. Soon you will notice intrusive thoughts and other sensations that distract you from attending fully to your breath. Your racing mind wants to take over, but resist the urge, and return to your breath.

4) When you are distracted by thoughts and other sensations, gently let them go. Do not dwell on them as you usually do. Return your attention to your breath. Also, avoid struggling with the thoughts. Do not try to get rid of them, as you often do when the thoughts are unpleasant. Simply acknowledge their presence and continue following your breath.

Practice this procedure every day to make it a habit. You can begin with a five-minute practice and gradually extend the time as you become more comfortable with it. You can do this exercise at any time and in any place for brief periods, especially when you are feeling depressed.

One word of caution. If you were traumatized as a child by abuse, being quiet and still may be overwhelming for you. Flashbacks and painful thoughts and feelings may emerge. Stop the practice if you feel overwhelmed. Learn your zone of tolerance and gradually incorporate quiet into your life.

In the second step, you continue the effort to know yourself. You sense that beneath the painful façade of your depressed mood is an unacknowledged strength. That strength comes from a Power greater than your depressed self, a Power that is both within and beyond you. It radiates from your neglected true, sane self.

Dennis Ortman, Ph.D.

Choose Life
Taking a Leap

Step three: "Made a decision to turn our will and our lives
over to the care of God as we understood Him."

"Every particle of creation sings its own song of what is and what is not.
Hearing what is can make you wise;
hearing what is not can drive you mad."

—Ghalib

You have entered the dark forest. Still, you hesitate to move forward. Only the distant light gives you enough hope and courage to fight your fear. You imagine a bright sun-like Source, even though all you see are faint glimmers. Cautiously, you begin to walk toward the Source of the light. It is your only guide through the darkness. You feel lost in that shadowy world. The path is treacherous, winding, with many holes and rocks to stumble on. You walk with one eye on the path and the other on the light.

In the previous Steps, you reflected on your depressing situation. You came to some understanding and acceptance of your powerlessness over your mood and your need to believe in a Power greater than yourself. Step three is the action step. You make the decision about who or what you want to believe in. In making that decision, you confront your self-will to control and your need for willingness to surrender.

LISTEN TO YOURSELF

Your depression interferes with your ability to think clearly, and you get caught in mental ruts. Making even small decisions can feel overwhelming. How can you make the life-changing decision to believe?

Angela, unable to think clearly:

"I walk around in a fog all day, like I'm asleep. My husband gets frustrated a lot because he has to repeat himself. He says I'm not paying attention. I can't help it. When I'm in a funk, I have a cotton brain. I can't concentrate or remember anything. When somebody even asks me what I want for dinner, I feel too confused to make up my mind. Sometimes I just break into tears because I'm so frustrated with myself."

Richard, caught in a mental rut:

"My son just lost his job and is having financial problems. I really want to help him, but I'm on a fixed income. I feel so guilty that I can't give him any money. What kind of father am I? I feel like I failed my son his whole life. I was never a good enough provider. I never taught him a good work ethic. His being fired is my fault because I didn't alert him to the dangers I saw on his job. My wife tells me I take on too much responsibility for other's problems. She's right. I guess there's no end to my self-blame."

To make a decision of faith, you need to find a way to calm your agitated mind. In your pessimism, you may not think that is possible. However, your black mood may encourage you to become a contemplative person. When depressed, you want to hibernate. You naturally withdraw from life to nurse your wounds. You disengage from the world, lacking energy or motivation for any involvement. The danger, of course, is that you can become lost in your obsessive negative thinking. Nevertheless, your withdrawal presents an opportunity to confront your confused and biased thoughts. You can learn to enter the stillness and quiet of your mood to discover hidden treasures. Your painful longing can open your heart to seek that treasure in God.

You can find what you seek so desperately by looking deeply within yourself, rather than outside yourself. That is the secret to an authentic, life-changing faith. As the Buddha taught in the *Kalamas Sutra*:

Do not believe in what you have heard; do not believe in traditions because they have been handed down for many generations; do not believe in anything because it was rumored and spoken by many; do not believe merely because the written statement of some old sage is produced; do not believe in conjectures; do not believe merely in the authority of your teachers and elders. After observation and analysis, when it agrees with reason and it is conducive to the good and benefit of one and all, then accept it and live up to it.

There is a temptation to follow the easy path and simply accept blindly your inherited religious tradition. Then your belief can become stale and superficial. Unfortunately, religion is often identified with conformity and control. Genuine faith seeks freedom and life. The third step invites you to pursue the narrow path of the founders of the great religions. Moses, Jesus, and Mohammed went out into the desert to be away from the crowd to fast and pray. Buddha went into the forest to meditate. In their stillness and solitude, they experienced a sacred Presence and made a life-changing choice.

CIRCUS OF THE MIND

Like all addictions, depression is fundamentally a disease of the mind. "Stinking thinking" rules you. Modern psychology affirms the power of the mind to influence feelings and behaviors. It echoes what the Buddha taught in his own common sense way 2600 years ago: "The mind is everything. What you think you become." It also resonates with Jesus' message: "Reform your lives and believe in the good news." The Greek word for "reform your lives" is *metanoia,* which literally means "change your mind." You can change your life by changing your mind and facing your tendency to hear only bad news.

In the grip of gloom, your own thinking persecutes you. You believe the world corresponds exactly to your thoughts about it. Because you think something, you believe it must be true, a fact of life. It never occurs to you how biased you are in your thinking. You also fail to realize how your self-centeredness makes you cling to your opinions, unwilling to let them go.

I attempt to nudge my patients out of their straightjacket thinking. I refer to their thoughts as "clouds," "mist," or "thought bubbles," suggesting their lightness and elusiveness. Many of my patients can admit that their feelings come and go, but they experience their thoughts as solid, steady, and reliable. They imagine their thoughts are the solid ground on which they stand.

A FOUR STEP PROCESS

To turn your will and life over, you need to change your mind. I recommend a four step process to help loosen the grip of your biased, pessimistic thinking. Because your thinking can become so entrenched, it will require determination, effort, and perseverance to change your mind.

1) Watch the parade.

First, become an observer of the free flow of your thoughts. Notice how the thoughts arise from nowhere and nothingness, pass through your mind, and return to emptiness. Have you ever asked yourself, "Where do my thoughts come from, and where do they go?" Recognize the almost steady stream of thoughts through your consciousness.

If you pay close attention, you will see gaps in the parade of changing thoughts. You cannot think about more than one thing at once, so your mind is constantly shifting. There is a brief pause as the mind shifts gears. The pause between the march of thoughts reveals your pure consciousness, which is the source of your thinking. You cannot observe that mindful awareness directly because there is no place to stand to view it. However, you can perceive its products in your thoughts. You can also sense the unbounded depth of the consciousness in experiencing the gaps.

You are probably so accustomed to being depressed, that you do not notice the automatic and repetitive thoughts that run through your mind. Pay close attention to the thoughts that arise from your depressed mind. If you do, over time, you will begin to notice a particular quality of thinking. You will begin to sense that you are being possessed by a mind of disappointment. That mind:

- is sensitive to losses and endings.

- focuses on how reality fails to meet your expectations.

- engages in scarcity thinking—there is never enough.

- is preoccupied with what is missing from the past.

As an observer, you will also notice that there is another mind beneath your superficial pessimistic thinking. That mind allows you to be an observer of yourself and others. It is the pure consciousness that dwells in the gaps of the parade of thoughts. I call it the mind of abundance that emerges from your true self, not your child-like depressed self, and connects you with all of reality. It enables you to see life from a larger perspective. The mind of abundance:

- embraces the fullness of experience, excluding nothing.

- focuses on what life offers, the gifts received.

- engages in abundance thinking—there is more than enough.

- dwells in the present moment on what is.

You will also note the constant interplay of the two minds. For all of us, to some degree, they are in continuous dialogue. Sometimes one mind is louder than the other and in control of your thinking in that moment. Notice who is talking at any particular moment.

2) Enjoy the circus.

Secondly, accept your conflicting minds and thoughts. Enjoy them. Your tendency is to be preoccupied with your negative thoughts and engage in a full-tilt battle to eliminate them. You try to ignore the thoughts, but they refuse to go away. You may distract yourself with activities, but the negative buzz persists. You may even attempt to replace the negative thoughts with positive ones. However, the unpleasant thoughts creep back into your mind, and may even grow in intensity.

Instead of fight or flight, I recommend that you embrace the mind of disappointment with love, and attempt to learn its wisdom. Enjoy the circus play of ideas. Remember that sadness is a natural emotion. It opens your heart to compassion. It alerts you to deeper unfulfilled longings. However, the noise of gloom may become so loud that it drowns out the voice of abundance, of good and plenty.

Depression, sensitive to darkness, can open you to the mystery of life beyond control and comprehension.

3) Appreciate the show.

Thirdly, investigate and try to understand your mind of disappointment. In talking about their depressed ideas, I tell my patients, "That's an interesting way of thinking. How did you learn to think that way?" Then, together, we investigate the history of each idea and way of thinking, tracing it back to its roots. Often, my patients echo the gloom of their parents. Parents pass on negative messages and styles of thinking to their children like a contagious disease. I suggest to my patients that their parents' thinking is only one possibility and that there are many alternatives. "It is really child-like thinking to hang on to something you learned from your parents as the truth," I tell them.

Investigating the depressing thoughts, you realize their persistence. You blindly accepted the same beliefs as absolute truth for a long time. Your opinions about reality become fixed and automatic, and you willfully hang on to them. Perhaps it never occurs to you how much faith you put into your own ideas of reality. You never question your views, only assume their accuracy. They give you a sense of security, "a still point in the turning world." Overwhelmed by the changes in your life, you crave the illusionary stability of fixed ideas and beliefs.

You also notice how indulging the mind of disappointment leads to depression, holding back, and suffering. The abundance thinking inspires gratitude, generosity, and happiness.

4) Follow the ringmaster.

Finally, listen to your mind of abundance. It is the reliable ringmaster that directs the show. It reflects mature thinking. See what makes sense to you in the cacophony of your pessimistic thoughts. Standing back, you can analyze and evaluate your depressing thoughts and beliefs. Do they make sense to you now? Are losses and fears being exaggerated? Are there blessings you ignore? Do you want to use those thoughts as a guide for action? What can you learn about yourself and your experience now? What unrealistic expectations do you hold about life? Observing and questioning the flow of your thoughts helps you to see their lightness and not give them so much weight. Furthermore, it helps you not to identify with your thoughts, making them the reality of who you are.

Your thoughts flow like a river that cannot be dammed up effectively. As much as you want to eliminate those unpleasant thoughts, all your efforts to do so will fail. However, you do have freedom to choose, with your mature mind, how much weight you give to those depressing thoughts. You are always free to choose how to behave, whether or not to act on those urges.

STEPS TO FREEING YOUR DEPRESSED MIND

1. Watch the parade: observe the flow of your thoughts.

2. Enjoy the circus: accept your conflicting minds and thoughts.

3. Appreciate the show: investigate your mind of disappointment.

4. Follow the ringmaster: listen to your mind of abundance.

Your depressed mood both inhibits and stimulates your decision of faith, your willingness to believe. You are exquisitely sensitive to the unknown in your life. You also know powerlessness intimately. Your sense of powerlessness and darkness may paralyze you. Or it may bring you to an encounter with the aura of mystery that surrounds you.

SWEET SURRENDER

Alcoholics Anonymous identifies in no uncertain terms the root cause of the addict's problems: "Our whole trouble had been the misuse of willpower...Step Three calls for affirmative action, for it is only by action that we cut away the self-will which has always blocked the entry of God—or, if you like, a Higher Power—into our lives" (1). Not trusting in anyone or anything but themselves, alcoholics try to control their moods, environment, and others with their drug. They firmly believe that their drug of choice will bring them happiness. Despite all the contrary evidence, they cling to that belief.

In your depression, you exhibit a will to power contrary to your sense of helplessness. You feel controlled by your moods. However, if you look more closely at your condition, you observe that your mood arises from your pessimistic thinking, which has become fixed. A set of rigid beliefs underlies that thinking. You hold those beliefs with an unmovable stubbornness. You profess that you are worthless, guilty, helpless, and hopeless. No one can convince you otherwise. You profess your faith in:

- Worthlessness: "I'm a defective person. Whenever someone compliments me, I don't believe it. When they criticize me, it confirms what I believe about myself. I get exhausted trying to prove my worth, but know I'll never succeed. No one could ever love me because I'm so unlovable."

- Guilt: "I bear full responsibility for myself and those I love. Whenever anything goes wrong, I blame myself. If something goes right, it's just blind luck. I try to do my best, but it is never good enough. I only deserve punishment for all my failures."

- Helplessness: "'I can't' is my middle name. I feel so inadequate. I've failed so often in my life that I now give up trying. It won't make any difference anyway."

- Hopelessness: "Everything has gone wrong in my life so far. I see no reason that the future will be any different. What is the meaning of it all? What purpose is there in living if all I experience is pain?"

Your image of God may match your self-image.

Emily, believing in a punishing God:

"Both my parents and my church taught me to be afraid. God was like a mean Santa Claus because I was told so often, 'You better watch out, you better not cry.' The sermons at church always reminded me that I was a sinner, that God was there judging me. I didn't need that reminder. I was a harsh enough judge of myself, my own worst critic. I was always waiting for some punishment, thinking I deserved it. When the pastor spoke about God's mercy, I just couldn't believe it."

You hold these beliefs with an unshakable faith. No one can convince you otherwise. Friends and family try to persuade you to be easier on yourself, but you resist their reassurances. They offer evidence of your goodness, but you reject it, insisting on your unworthiness. You may recognize that these beliefs cause you terrible emotional pain, but you still hang on to them.

What purpose could these pessimistic beliefs serve? Change overwhelms you. These firm beliefs, even though distorted, provide you with the illusion of stability in your topsy-turvy world. You can tell yourself, with an air of certainty, "This I know to be true!"

There is a key to unlock you from your mental prison of negativity. The key is willingness. It opens the door for you to experience your life fully and let the awareness of God enter it. Locked into your depression, you cling to many ideas that suck the life out of you. All you need to do is surrender those entrenched thoughts and beliefs. Then you can freely enter your experience. You can choose life.

When we uncover these hidden beliefs in therapy, I invite my patients to consider some questions. I comment, "That's an interesting way to view yourself. How did you come to think that way? What purpose could it serve for you to see yourself so negatively? Could there be another way of looking at yourself that would be more beneficial?"

NAME YOUR GOD

The third step invites you to be a theologian. Based on your personal experience, it asks you to answer the question, "What is my ultimate concern?" Whatever is ultimate for you becomes your God. Coming to faith, you naturally seek to name and learn about your God. Faith seeks understanding. The third step encourages you to undertake an intelligent personal search for your God. It also reminds you of the gap between the reality of God and your thoughts about Him.

All religious traditions underline the Mystery of the Divine, the gap that can only be bridged by faith. The *Tao Te Ching* teaches in the opening verse: "The tao (God) that can be told is not the eternal Tao (God), the name that can be named is not the eternal Name." Whatever we think or say about God does not adequately reflect the fullness of His reality. Buddhists remind us that all our talk about ultimate Reality, "is not the moon, only a finger pointing to the moon." Saint Paul instructs, "Now we are seeing a dim reflection in a mirror; but then we shall be seeing face to face" (I Cor 13:12). We approach the Divine Mystery with humility, acknowledging the limitations of our understanding.

T.S. Elliot expresses the proper attitude in approaching this Mystery: "There are only hints and guesses, hints followed by guesses; and the rest is prayer, observance, discipline, thought and action" (2). As much as you want assurance of the rightness of your faith, there are no guarantees. You cannot prove that you are right and another wrong in their beliefs. God is infinitely larger than your ideas about Him. The only indication of the sincerity and rightness of your faith in your God is how it affects your living. The God you choose to believe in must inspire you toward growth and working the Steps.

Your concern is not simply whether or not God exists. You want to know the disposition of the Divine toward you before you are ready to put yourself in His care. Do you see God as benevolent, malevolent, or uninvolved? For you or against you? Can you place all your trust in this God?

WHO: PUNISHING OR FORGIVING GOD?

Recent research shows that Americans think differently about God. Ninety two percent claim that they believe in God. However, the ways they think about the Divinity vary.

Sixty percent view God as a Person, while twenty five percent consider God an impersonal force in the universe. Seven percent say it is impossible to know anything about God (3).

Among all these religious opinions, who is right? Is God a personal Being, an impersonal force, unknowable, or nonexistent? Each of us answer that question for ourselves. For those who choose to believe, no explanation is necessary. For those who choose not to believe, no explanation is possible. Furthermore, how we think about God cannot be verified as either true or false. Talking about God is similar to discussing theories about light. We experience light, but are at a loss to define it adequately. Some view light as particles of photons, while others consider it a wave. God is beyond the personal and impersonal categories we use to describe our experience of Him/It.

Those who see God in personal terms perceive His character differently. A recent Baylor University study of college students (4) indicated that thirty one percent believed in an authoritarian God who is judging and wrathful. Twenty three percent professed faith in a benevolent, forgiving God. Sixteen percent viewed God as critical but just, while twenty four percent considered God distant, uninvolved.

Your depression may condition you to form an image of God that matches your negative self-image. What you believe about yourself becomes transferred to God. You see yourself as a defective, fallen person. You judge yourself harshly, expecting punishment. So you imagine yourself a sinner in the hands of an angry God. You see God as a harsh Judge who punishes severely with hell fire. Such pessimistic faith will likely reinforce your depressed mood.

Another view of God and yourself may be more beneficial in your recovery. You can see yourself and God in more positive terms. The Bible also presents God as a loving Father and all of us as His beloved children. He forgives sins and desires our happiness. Imagining yourself as a child embraced by a loving, forgiving God will more likely inspire you to work at your recovery.

WHAT: HOSTILE OR FRIENDLY UNIVERSE?

Bill Wilson, the cofounder of Alcoholics Anonymous thought of God in impersonal terms:

> *"The word God still aroused a certain antipathy. When the thought was expressed that there might be a God personal to me, this feeling intensified. I didn't like the idea. I could go for such conceptions as Creative Intelligence, Universal Mind or Spirit of Nature, but I resisted the thought of a Czar of the Heavens, however loving His sway might be. I have since talked with scores of men who felt the same way"* (5).

A majority of the original members of the AA fellowship were agnostics or atheists who struggled to find faith. Like Bill Wilson and his friends, you may find the idea of God presented in personal terms suspect. You are aware of the danger of creating God in your own image and likeness, rather than the other way around. Such a subjective view of God holds little weight for you. Furthermore, you may object to the idea of a Supreme Being in the heavens, apart from, overseeing, and controlling the world. He is too disengaged.

If you are of a more scientific-minded temperament, you may prefer to view God as an Intelligence or Life Force more intimately involved in the workings of the world. The energy and Spirit of such a God also pervades all creation, including you and your fellow human beings. As the poet Dylan Thomas wrote, "The force that through the green fuse drives the flower drives my green age."

To entrust yourself to the care of an impersonal God, you need to address the question that Einstein poses: "The most important decision we make is whether we believe in a friendly or hostile universe." There is no rational proof, but plenty of evidence to support either choice. Believing the universe is hostile encourages pessimism, paranoia, and despair about life. Believing in its friendliness inspires optimism, openness, and joy. It also inspires confidence in your own goodness.

PARADOX OF SURRENDER AND VICTORY

"I did it my way," Frank Sinatra famously sang. That is also our natural instinct. Taking charge of your life displays your strength of character, your determination, your will power. The third step may shock you in its recommendation to exchange willfulness for willingness, to turn your life and will over to another. You may protest, "That's submission, allowing another to dominate me. I won't tolerate that!"

The third step proposes a surprising paradox for recovery: "We surrender to win." What do we surrender and what do we win? When you work the third step, you give up your self-centered ways of thinking and believing that reinforce your depressed mood. You gain a sense of freedom to be yourself.

Your natural instinct is to battle against your depressed feelings because they are so painful. However, if you work so hard to get rid of them, you may miss their wisdom. The third step encourages you to surrender to the mood and embrace it fully. Lean into it, rather than against it, to learn its message. Underlying the mood are fixed ideas and beliefs about yourself and life, and a longing for meaning and wholeness. Allow yourself to be aware of these silent assumptions. See them for the empty, passing thoughts that they are. Then, let them go. Surrender them, instead of hanging on to them as firm truths. In the process, you will gain a victory. You will release God's Power within you, which enables you to be yourself.

HOW: INSIGHT MEDITATION EXERCISE

When you are depressed, either a brain fog or jumbled thoughts of catastrophic losses occupy you. Such thoughts keep you on edge and prevent you from seeing yourself and the world accurately. Lost in your thoughts, you remain on the surface of life. Its abundance eludes you.

A traditional eastern practice called Vipassana, which means "insight meditation," can help you listen to the wondrous depths of your own consciousness. It is sometimes called "choiceless awareness" or "bare awareness" (6). The purpose of the exercise is to help you connect with the vast openness of your consciousness. The procedure for this practice is simple, similar to the exercise of following your breath.

1) Find a quiet place. Assume a relaxed posture, with your back straight and head erect. You may sit on a chair with your feet on the floor, or on a cushion in the lotus position. Place your hands on your lap with the palms facing up in a receptive position. Keep your eyes open, focused on a spot in front of you.

2) Breathe deeply from your abdomen and follow your breath, as in the previous exercise. Feel the air filling the various parts of your body, relaxing all the tension in your muscles.

3) Begin with the conscious intention to be open to whatever arises in your consciousness. Welcome everything, the delightful and the unpleasant. Make the intention not to judge or reject whatever you experience.

4) As you quiet your mind and relax your body, notice the various thoughts, feelings, and sensations that arise. Note them and gently let go of them. Returning to your breath can help you hold the contents of your consciousness lightly. Just be an observer of all that comes and goes through your mind. Also pay attention to your spontaneous emotional reactions to the contents, whether you like, dislike, or are neutral to what you perceive. Notice what persists and tends to grab on to your awareness. Let that go also.

5) As you observe the flow of your consciousness, you can make a mental note of what you experience. Simply label a thought, feeling, or sensation, saying to yourself, "thought," "feeling," or "sensation." Do not ponder what you observe at this time.

6) After the meditation, take a few minutes to reflect on what you experienced. Take note of any powerful and repeating thoughts, feelings, and sensations.

Make this practice a daily habit, alternating it with the practice of following your breath. If the practice raises overwhelming traumatic memories, stop until you are ready. Begin with a fifteen minute meditation and extend the time as you become more adept. Remember, practice does not make perfect, but makes progress.

In the third step, you make a conscious decision to believe. You begin the lifelong process of surrendering your self-centered will and opening yourself to let the Power of God work through you.

9

Night Vision
An Honest Look

Step Four: "Made a searching and fearless moral inventory of ourselves."

"If you realize that all things change,
There is nothing you will try to hold on to."

—Lao-tzu

You proceed deeper into the forest, following the distant light. The light fades and reappears, provoking alternating dread and fear in you. The path winds, like a labyrinth. You walk cautiously to avoid falling into the holes and getting mired in the muck. A strange thing happens as the distant light intensifies. The shadows that surround you become more threatening. They take the shapes of wild beasts and demons. In your terror, you wonder to yourself, "How could I have been so foolish to venture into this forest?" You tense yourself for battle, thinking, "I'd better kill them before they kill me!"

In the fourth step, you begin the process of cleaning house. The process involves taking an honest look at yourself, warts and all. To undertake such an investigation requires humility, honesty, and courage. Unless you have taken the three previous Steps, you will not be able to muster the courage to look and see yourself clearly. Unless you have some faith in God, a Higher Power, or Ultimate Reality and see your life from a larger perspective, your self-searching will hit a wall. What you glimpse may discourage you.

You may wonder to yourself, "What needs to be cleaned up?" You want to wipe away your depressed mood, which creates a mess with your life. You want it cleaned up now, not later, because of all the pain it causes you. However, the fourth step invites you to stay with the pain and learn the message of your mood. Your depression is not your real problem, as you imagine, but the symptom of a deeper problem you need to explore.

Alcoholics Anonymous alerts you to the core of your problem: "Nearly every serious emotional problem can be seen as a case of misdirected instinct. When that happens, our great natural assets, the instincts, have been turned into physical and mental liabilities" (1). Some hidden desires, pursued with reckless abandon, give rise to your depression. Their pursuit knocks you off balance and keeps you from your journey home to your true self.

How can you uncover these misdirected instincts? That is the work of the Steps. The *Tao Te Ching*, referring to qualities of a great nation and great person, expresses clearly and concisely the steps of housecleaning:

> **When he makes a mistake he realizes it.**
> **Having realized it, he admits it.**
> **Having admitted it, he corrects it (61).**

In step four, you begin the process of realizing your mistakes and untangling yourself. In step five you admit them to another. Then, in Steps six through nine, you work at correcting them.

OBSTACLES TO SOUL-SEARCHING

Realizing your mistakes requires humility, which is truth. Humility means seeing yourself as you really are, not as you wish to be. This honest self-examination involves walking a difficult middle path between denial and self-loathing. The biggest obstacle to this soul-searching is pride, your desire to be perfect. That perfectionism represents a secret desire to be God, all-knowing and all-powerful. The Steps/Traditions book warns: "This perverse soul-sickness is not pleasant to look at. Instincts on rampage balk at investigation" (p. 44).

Pride shows itself in two opposing ways: as ego-inflation and ego-deflation. You think of yourself as more or less than you really are. The first way may surprise you, and the second is all too familiar to you in your depression.

Rebecca, the judge:

> *"I became a lawyer because I love to argue and win. I have to be right and do not hesitate to fight for what I believe in. My parents noticed that in me and always told me I would be a great lawyer. They were right. I had a very successful career as an attorney, but realized my dream when I was elected to be a judge in the District Court. I had arrived. It thrills me to hear cases, listen to all the opposing arguments, and then make my decision. My word is final. I have the last word, always."*

If you tend to see yourself as more than you are, you make yourself a hero in your inner narrative. You cultivate an inflated self-image. In your own mind, you are an important, special person. Holding high standards for yourself and others, you relish the pursuit of these ideals. Because of your accomplishments, you feel superior to others. You enjoy their esteem and admiration. Their criticism may sting you, but you learn to ignore it. You may admit some minor faults, but you imagine that your special character more than makes up for them. Self-satisfied, no one can stand in your way on your heroic journey to perfection. You tell yourself, "I can't do anything wrong."

While you acknowledge your strengths, you fail to recognize and acknowledge your weaknesses. Your proud arrogance is an exaggeration of healthy self-esteem. Your inflated self-worth actually hides a deep-seated sense of unworthiness. You feel needy and unlovable, but cannot bear seeing it yourself or allowing others to see it. So you hide behind a mask of perfection. Secretly, you know you are not living up to your high standards and feel depressed about it.

Ann Marie, the housewife:

"I'm a stay-at-home mom. My husband and I agreed that I would not work and would stay home to take care of the kids. I know it's an important job to be a mother, but I still feel something is missing in my life. I envy other mothers who can balance work and home. I'm just not strong or smart enough to do both. I'm so lazy. My husband works long hours. I don't feel like I'm contributing my fair share."

If you tend to see yourself as less than you are, you make yourself a loser in your personal drama. You nurture a deflated self-image. Constantly comparing yourself to others, you see yourself as inferior. Others accomplish so much more than you in your mind. You feel like a failure, even though you cannot articulate clearly the standards by which you judge yourself. Nevertheless, you are a judge who shows no mercy to yourself. You constantly feel guilty and indulge in self-pity. You tell yourself, "I can't do anything right."

While you acknowledge your weaknesses, you fail to recognize your strengths. You paint a black and white picture of yourself, but the dark overshadows the light. Your harsh self-criticism is really an exaggerated modesty. It hides an underlying pride. In reality, you entertain high standards and long for perfection. But you can never live up to those hidden expectations about yourself. You live with a constant sense of not being good enough.

Emotions Anonymous expresses clearly the consequences of these high expectations on your moods: "In our search for self-worth and identity, we may have unknowingly set unrealistic goals for ourselves. Because our ideals are too high and we can never live up to these unrealistic expectations, our sense of self-worth is low. How can we but fail?" (p.17). The gap between your expectations and experience, between what you long for and what you get, results in a painful sense of loss and a depressed mood.

MORAL INVENTORY: EXPOSING THE HIDDEN

You may wonder, "Why do I need a moral inventory?" Unlike someone addicted to alcohol or drugs, who appears to choose to use, you had no choice about being depressed. You may believe you were born with this condition, and wish you were not. You see yourself as a victim suffering many losses. Your moods possess you against your will. You feel powerless over them.

Behind your depressed reaction, however, lurk many unacknowledged attachments, hidden cravings that throw your life out of balance. You lost something important. You protest the imposed, unwanted change. Distressed by your ever-changing life with unavoidable losses, you hang on desperately to some fixed ideas about the way to happiness. You look for a "still point in the turning world." Your depression expresses hidden desires, frozen still points, which are unconscious choices regarding value for you.

How do you clean house? How do you discover your secret cravings beneath your mood?

PAY ATTENTION TO YOUR FEELINGS

When depressed, you have three natural reactions to your painful mood. First, you fight against the sadness and engage in self-criticism. "I don't want to feel this way. I shouldn't feel this way," you tell yourself. You may then become impatient with yourself, judging yourself a failure because you cannot make the sadness go away. You may come to believe you are defective because the uncomfortable feelings persist. Secondly, you attempt to flee the feeling by distracting yourself. If you ignore it, you hope it will go away. "This is just a passing sadness," you tell yourself. Finally, you freeze into the feeling, allowing it to absorb you. All you think about is your pain and sorrow.

I recommend that you become an astute and compassionate observer of your depressed mood. Contrary to your natural instincts, lean into and relax into the mood. Soften your body and let go of the tension you feel. Allow yourself to feel deeply the sadness at what you have lost. Immerse yourself into the feeling. Notice where in your body you hold the pain: a heavy heart, an upset stomach, a restless body. Take note of the quality of the mood: the intensity, the frequency, the pattern of its ebb and flow. Observe the rising and falling of the mood. Pay attention to the events that trigger your sad reaction, the losses to which you are most sensitive. Then notice how you react to your uncomfortable feelings: by fighting, fleeing, or freezing.

Next, extend kindness and compassion to yourself in your suffering. Instead of viewing your depression as an enemy, consciously choose to see it as a friend. Welcome the feeling with an open mind and heart. You may see yourself possessed by the mood. Begin to heal the division within yourself with a wholehearted acceptance of what you do not like within yourself. Assume the attitude of Jesus and Buddha when they encountered their demons. Jesus made an effort to get to know the names of the devils he cast out. Buddha invited the demons for tea so he could get better acquainted with them. Befriend your feelings so you can learn from them.

Thirdly, investigate carefully what your feeling is trying to tell you. Listen closely to your depressed feeling to learn its wisdom. Sadness, sorrow, and depression are natural re-actions to loss. Probe, with your open, nonjudgmental mind, what you are missing in your life. Notice the deeper feelings within the feeling. What do you want that you are not get-ting? How do you feel about not getting it—angry, envious, self-pitying, etc.? In what are you disappointed? What expectations about yourself and others are not being met? Your sadness reveals your unique sensitivities and what you hang on to for security and comfort. Notice what triggers your mood and what you tend to obsess about.

Finally, do not identify with your mood. Your feelings come from you, but they are not you. You are the blue sky, while your feelings are passing clouds. The more you can become an observer of your feelings, the less you will identify with them. But it takes practice. You may say, "I'm a depressed person." However, your mood does not define you as a per-son. You may also say, "I'm feeling depressed." However, the feeling of the moment passes quickly and contains many other feelings. To be exact, you can tell yourself, "I'm having the feeling that I'm depressed." That is closer to the truth for your experience in the moment.

You react with sadness when you lose something you want. Understanding your sorrowful reactions can help you discover your hidden desires.

PEEL THE ONION

There are many layers to your depressed mood that you may not readily recognize. Your depression reveals your longing for wholeness and where you are stuck. You become stuck when you cling to some desire, some fixed belief, and try to make it the whole of your life. Your depressed mood cries out in protest. It tells you that some instinct is out of balance with your life. What you are depressed about having lost reveals what you are hanging on to too tightly.

Bill Wilson, the cofounder of AA, considered himself a hopeless drunk. He tried many times to stop, but relapsed regularly. He also suffered from severe depression. Several times he was suicidal and hospitalized. The depression and drinking worked in tandem, causing him to spiral out of control. Despite his best efforts, he could find no relief from his depression or drinking. A breakthrough came, however, when he realized he had another unacknowledged addiction. He desperately needed praise and approval from others. Approval became his drug. Only when he addressed this addiction was he able to achieve emotional sobriety.

Like Bill Wilson, you may uncover many layers to your mood. Each layer reveals a new challenge.

Joseph, lost in grief:

"When my wife Bernie died, my life fell apart. I thought about committing suicide because I had no reason to live. I wanted to be with her. I didn't believe I could survive on my own. Thank God I found an understanding therapist who helped me through my grief. I learned so much about myself. I never realized how dependent I had become on Bernie in every area of my life. I had no life of my own. My depression challenged me to build a new life for myself, to become an independent person."

Nathan, desperately wanting approval:

"From as far back as I can remember, I wanted to please my father. But he was a man who could not be satisfied. Anything I did was not good enough. I became so depressed that one day I decided to kill myself by taking pills. Fortunately, my parents found me before it was too late and took me to the hospital. That was so crazy. I was willing to die because I didn't have my father's approval."

The following are some typical sticking points you may discover as you peel away the skins of your depression. Reflect on what you lost when you became depressed.

"I became depressed when my boyfriend left me." You will naturally grieve for a while after the breakup of a relationship with someone you care about. However, you may become obsessed with the lost love. You may believe you need to be loved by that person to be happy. You may have become addicted to love without realizing it.

"I became depressed when my children left home." The empty nest syndrome challenges you to develop a new life for yourself. After devoting yourself to caring for your children, you may have lost yourself in your parental role. You realize your need to be needed. It dawns on you how much your self-esteem is dependent on being recognized for helping others.

"I became depressed when I was fired from my job." A man's identity in our society is closely connected with his work and performance. The job loss awakens you to your excessive need to succeed. Success also brought you the approval from others you crave. You came to believe that you must accumulate achievements to be fulfilled as a person.

"I became depressed when my boss corrected me for making a mistake." The intensity of the feelings of humiliation may have surprised you. You naturally want to defend yourself and your position. The correction may awaken in you an awareness of the strength of your needs to be right and to look good.

"I became depressed when my close friend criticized me." When you are criticized you feel like a total failure. In your mind, either you are perfect or you are worthless. The need to be perfect may be overwhelming for you, causing you to push yourself relentlessly. Any imperfection enrages you. There is a lot at stake for you. You believe you have to be perfect to be accepted by others.

"I became depressed when I got seriously ill." If your life has been devoted to seeking happiness and avoiding pain, a serious illness can be devastating. The loss of your health creates intolerable suffering. You live with the illusion that you can create a life for yourself without pain.

"I became depressed when the demands of my life became too much for me." You may coast through life, avoiding as much stress as possible. When unexpected challenges happen, you may be easily overwhelmed and want to give up. In those moments you realize the power of your need for peace and quiet.

"I became depressed when I did not get what I wanted from my spouse." You may entertain high expectations for yourself and others, which you do not clearly recognize. When those expectations are not met, you become disappointed. Over time, the disappointment changes into resentment.

FROM SHAME TO GUILT

You may feel ashamed about being depressed and want to hide it from others. You imagine that others see you as inferior, weak, and defective because you are depressed. There is a stigma about mental illness in our society. That prejudice is born of fear and ignorance. The mind is so mysterious, and the darkness within so frightening. You may share that prejudice and think of yourself in only negative terms. That gives you a reason to attack yourself for any mistakes or flaws. You can be merciless in those attacks, imagining that all you deserve is punishment.

Shame interferes with your ability to make an honest self-assessment. While in the trance of unworthiness, all you can see are your defects. You likely exaggerate them. Then, taking an inventory only becomes an exercise in humiliation, not true humility.

To make an honest moral inventory, you need to transform your shame into a healthy guilt, measuring yourself against realistic standards. Shame announces, "I am a mistake."

Guilt says, "I made a mistake." Shame identifies the sinner with the sin, while guilt can separate the two. When you have a healthy sense of guilt for wrongdoing, you tell yourself, "I'm better than that behavior."

Seeing yourself more clearly, you acknowledge your basic goodness and have realistic standards of excellence. You are able to stand back and assess how well you live up to those standards. You take full responsibility for your behavior. When you fail, you do not just beat yourself up. You feel remorse. Your remorse motivates you to change the behavior and move on. The guilty feeling does not linger.

When something unpleasant happens, my depressed patients say, "I feel bad. It is all my fault." They automatically blame themselves for anything that goes wrong in their lives. I invite them to stop and think, engaging their mature, rational mind. I ask, "What are you guilty of? What moral standard did you violate?" I encourage them to confront their shame-based self-centeredness and recognize the limits of their responsibility.

LOOK TO OTHERS

The more we get to know ourselves, the more we appreciate our depth and richness. There is more to us than we know. We never cease to amaze ourselves at the unexpected thoughts, reactions, and behaviors that come from us. Psychologists label it the unconscious. Like an iceberg, our conscious life is only the ten percent above the water, while the rest is yet unknown in the depths.

Self-reflection may not be enough to plumb your depths. Humbly aware of your limits, you do not need to rely on yourself alone for your moral inventory. You can learn from others. Certainly, you can get valuable feedback from those who love you. However, another resource for self-awareness is your critics and enemies. You can learn from them with the proper attitude. I have two suggestions.

First, welcome criticism and see your critics as teachers. The *Tao Te Ching* states, "(A great man) considers those who point out his faults as his most benevolent teachers" (61). You have blind spots, like everybody else. Your depressed mood makes you fearful to take off your blinders because you imagine you will see terrible things and feel worse about yourself. Those who criticize you can give you valuable feedback. They can give you a different perspective on yourself, letting you know how you come across to others. You might be surprised at what you hear if you are open.

Can criticism and correction really hurt you? Always evaluate what others say about you, weighing its truthfulness. Take what helps, and discard the rest. No one likes criticism. You may secretly yearn to be perfect. The criticism of others has power to disturb you to the extent that it echoes what you are already telling yourself. Your own inner critic is harsher than anything anyone else could tell you.

Secondly, see your enemy as your shadow. "(A great man) thinks of his enemy as the shadow that he himself casts," the *Tao Te Ching* (61) observes. To avoid looking honestly at yourself, you may turn your attention to the faults of others. You see the splinter in their eye, not the plank in your own. I encourage you to pay close attention to what you dislike in others, to what drives you crazy about them. Notice their annoying habits. However, instead of condemning them, ask yourself honestly if you can identify with any of those irritating behaviors. If you are honest with yourself, you will discover that what you hate in others, you despise and disown in yourself. In other words, if you spot it, you got it.

PARADOX OF SICKNESS AND HEALTH

Your depression confronts you with a paradox: "Through sickness we come to health." You can accept that you suffer the illness of depression and want it to end. You want symptom relief. In your haste, however, you avoid your deeper sickness of soul at the root of your mood. In reality, you will only become healthy when you are thoroughly sick of being sick.

What is sickness? When you are depressed, it is a sign that something is seriously out of balance in your life. The core of your being is crying out for attention. You are neglecting something that is essential for you to be fully alive. Your depression announces that you are dying inside because you are disconnected from the Source or your wellbeing. How are you disconnected? You are hanging on to something too tightly. Some loss has become intolerable to you. You hold on to that loss, even though it is killing your spirit. You may cling to the distorted belief that you cannot be happy without whatever you have lost.

Your depressed mood indicates that you are stuck in the flow of life. Your priorities are off and need to be reexamined. Your sickness invites you to explore more deeply what is missing in your life and what you truly value. Your loss of interest in your current life encourages you to be contemplative and find your true center, the Source. Only then will you restore balance to your life. Then you will feel alive and healthy.

PRACTICE: A MEDITATION ON SADNESS

Another practice to help you on the path toward self-awareness is meditating on select passages from the Bible. I suggest that you meditate on the following verses from the Gospel of Mark 10:17-22 (2). Jesus is addressing the rich young man, and you, personally. Consider the words a personal message from Jesus to you:

As Jesus was setting out on a journey a man came running up, knelt down before him and asked, "Good Teacher, what must I do to share in everlasting life?" Jesus answered, "Why do you call me good? No one is good but God alone. You know the commandments:

'You shall not kill.
You shall not commit adultery.
You shall not steal.
You shall not bear false witness.
You shall not defraud.
Honor your father and your mother.'"

He replied, "Teacher, I have kept all these since my childhood." Then Jesus looked at him with love and told him "There is one thing more you must do. Go and sell what you have and give it to the poor; you then will have treasure in heaven. After that, come and follow me." At these words the man's face fell. He went away sad, for he had many possessions.

The following steps summarize a meditation practice called, *lectio divina* (3), a divine reading:

1) Sit comfortably in a quiet place with your Bible. Take a few moments to quiet yourself and focus on being present in the moment. Be aware of God's presence and love for you. Ask Him to open your mind and heart to His words.

2) Read the words of the passage slowly. Allow the words to penetrate your soul. Imagine Jesus addressing you in your here-and-now situation with all your sadness. If a phrase jumps out at you, allow yourself to linger over it. Savor the phrase, taste its truth. Realize your own goodness and strength, like the rich young man who kept all the commandments. Then, reflect on your own sadness, which results from holding on too tightly to some distorted belief. What do you believe you must have to be happy, like the man who needed all his possessions? Consider your own personal list: perfection, approval, love, possessions, power, status, security, and so forth.

3) Next, respond spontaneously to the words. Let the feelings of gratitude at your abundance, or discouragement at your scarcity, emerge without hindering them. Reflect for a moment on your reactions to the words and what they reveal about you. Let your concerns show themselves.

4) After a time of reflection on the word and your reactions, rest in silence. Let all the chattering thoughts pass and do not dwell on them. Be still and sense God's loving presence. Enjoy the stillness and peace, which may be unfamiliar to you. The silence may be uncomfortable for you at the beginning. Stay with it. Extend the quiet time, from just a few minutes to as long as you like, as you become more familiar with this practice.

5) Finally, end the session with a spontaneous prayer of thanksgiving. Carry a meaningful phrase with you throughout the day.

The Twelve Steps flow in an alternating rhythm of contemplation and action. After taking your moral inventory, you prepare for action in the next step. What you learn about yourself you will share with another. Being honest with yourself, you can be truthful with others.

Dennis Ortman, Ph.D.

10

Lighten the Burden
Truth Telling

Step Five: "Admitted to God, to ourselves, and to another human being the exact nature of our wrongs."

"The only wisdom we can hope to acquire is the wisdom of humility: humility is endless."

—T.S. Eliot

Walking deeper into the woods, the shadows engulf you. The light remains your guide. It gives you courage to proceed. Glancing back, you see a larger shadow looming that frightens you. You run to escape it, stumbling over the rocks, holes, and fallen branches on the path. The shadow follows. You cannot escape it. Feeling alone, you shout out in terror, wishing someone would be there to accompany you on the journey. Suddenly, you recognize the shadow as your own.

In step five, your recovery takes an interpersonal turn. You spent time and effort getting to know your painful self, your higher self, and your shadow-self. The intimacy deepens when you share yourself with another. You get a response, feedback, and you see yourself through the mirror of another's reactions. As the *Tao Te Ching* teaches, admitting your mistakes furthers your personal house cleaning.

Commenting on step five, the Steps/Traditions book states: "All of AA's Twelve Steps ask us to go contrary to our natural desires...they all deflate our egos. When it comes to ego deflation, few Steps are harder to take than Five" (p. 55). Confessing faults to another is a humbling, ego-shattering experience. Your immediate reaction may be, "I don't need to feel any more deflated than I do!" So why do you need to take this step?

If you make a thorough moral inventory, it begins to dawn on you that you wear a mask of misery. Your depressed mood disguises a secret, hard-to-acknowledge need to be perfect. You wish to be special, loved by all, completely successful in everything you do, and beyond criticism or correction. In other words, you desire to be God. Of course, you cannot live up to those impossible standards and feel depressed about it.

This step sounds gloomy. You imagine it can only deepen your depression. Your ego seems deflated enough. However, avoiding this step and taking a short-cut will only keep you stuck in your mood and negative thinking. You need to go down into your depths before you can rise to new life.

You have already begun your downward journey. Admitting your powerlessness over your mood launched you on the path to recovery. That humbled you. This second admission is of your faults. This acknowledgment involves a deeper awareness and whole-hearted acceptance of your character defects. Telling another makes the faults more real and personal. You will only undertake the difficult work of correcting your faults when you see them in their naked truth.

HIDING

Sedated by your depression, you may hesitate to make this frank admission to another. Your sense of shame and need to withdraw interfere.

Rosemary, hiding her shame:

> *"I abused heroin when I was younger. Even though I've been clean for twenty years and turned my life around, I'm ashamed of my past. I hurt so many people I love. I have so many regrets and feel terrible about myself for what I did. I'm grateful that I now have a close relationship with my sons, but I'll never talk with them about the past. I just pretend that the craziness of my addiction never happened. They would probably forgive me, but I can't forgive myself."*

Another name for depression is low self-esteem. You judge yourself against your high standards and fail to measure up. Preoccupation with regrets and not being good enough take over your thoughts. You feel ashamed about what you did and also about who you are as a person. You believe you are defective. Shame reveals a false pride, a disappointment in yourself for not being perfect. You hang on to the regrets and refuse to forgive yourself. No wonder you want to hide.

Craig, withdrawing from life:

> *"When I get depressed, all I want to do is sleep. I don't want to see anyone or talk with anyone. I just want to be alone. It takes too much energy to be around people when I feel this way. I can't think clearly anyway. It takes too much effort to have even a simple conversation."*

When depressed, you feel drugged. Drained of energy and motivation, you want to disengage from life. You isolate yourself because you have no interest in being with others. Socializing requires too much effort. It is not that you enjoy your own company being alone. You hate your own life and do not want to be a burden to others. It is less trouble to be alone, so you hibernate.

CONFESSION

I was raised Catholic in the 1950s before the Second Vatican Council. I vividly remember my first confession in the second grade. It was a prerequisite before first communion. The nuns prepared us to examine our conscience in detail by measuring our lives against the Ten Commandments. They invited us to see how we failed in keeping God's rules and to keep an accurate count of the number of times we sinned. Going to confess to the priest was a terrifying experience. I entered a dark room, knelt down, and talked to the priest through a screen. I listed what I had done wrong and how many times. He absolved me and gave me a penance. The relief was in getting it over with and surviving.

My Protestant friends were baffled by the need for confession. They said, "Why can't you just talk to God directly? Why do you need to tell a priest?" My only answer was, "That's what we were taught. The nuns said it was tradition."

Since that time, I've learned more about the history and meaning of confession. In the first centuries of the Church, men and women chose to live in the desert to devote themselves entirely to prayer. They learned the benefit of revealing their faults to one another to gain insight and humility. The early Irish monks admitted their faults daily to their spiritual guides. They explored the roots of their motivations to become free of their influence. The practice spread throughout the whole Church. All the faithful were encouraged to confess their sins regularly to a priest to receive God's word of forgiveness.

After I was ordained a priest in 1975, my role expanded. Not only did I confess my sins to another, but I heard confessions. The Catholic world had changed by that time, after the winds of change from the Council blew through the Church. Few people went to confession in the old way. Some listed their sins in the semi-automatic way they learned as children. Others came less frequently, spoke from the heart, and unburdened their guilt.

Another change occurred in the practice. What we once called confession became known as the Sacrament of Reconciliation. Instead of a dark confessional box, people came into a bright, decorated reconciliation room where they had the choice to talk with the priest face-to-face. The atmosphere of the practice changed dramatically, from a preoccupation with guilt to a celebration of forgiveness. The rote listing of sins became a personal conversation. The frequency of confession decreased, while the intensity of the experience increased. It became more an experience of joy than dread.

Now, as a psychologist, I hear many confessions in my consultation room. My patients talk openly about their failings and their successes. Together, we explore what motivates their behavior and attempt to uncover the roots of their faults. My patients come to recognize their self-defeating behaviors and resolve to change their lives, allowing their true selves to emerge.

Alex, sexually abused as a child:

> *"I began therapy because I was feeling so depressed. I was unhappy with my life, but didn't exactly know the reason. I'd been molested by a male neighbor when I was very young, but never told anyone about it. I just stuffed it in the back of my mind. I*

figured it was the past and over with. One day, after two years of therapy, I decided to tell my therapist about the incident. I couldn't believe how nervous I felt, but I somehow knew I had to tell him about what happened. My therapist, a kind man, just listened. At the end of my story, he simply said, 'It wasn't your fault. You were just a child.' A great burden was lifted after that confession. I had secretly blamed myself all those years."

BENEFITS OF ADMITTING

You will never take the risk of revealing what you do not like about yourself unless you believe it will benefit you. Admitting your faults honestly, fearlessly, and humbly counterbalances your depressive tendencies and expands your consciousness. Admitting them will help you to:

- Overcome isolation.
- Receive acceptance.
- Experience humility.
- Confront self-deception.
- Show strength.
- Sense God's presence.

OVERCOME ISOLATION

The Steps/Traditions Book observes: "Almost without exception, alcoholics are tortured by loneliness...nearly all of us suffered the feeling that we didn't quite belong" (p. 57). The loneliness of the depressed matches that of the alcoholic. However, others do not cut you off because of your intolerable behavior, like happens to many alcoholics. You isolate yourself. Feeling unworthy and fatigued, you withdraw from the social arena. You lack the energy and self-esteem to interact with others.

The fifth step encourages you to move out of your isolation, not bearing the burden of your faults alone. As the AA saying goes, "If you share your pain, you cut it in half; if you don't, you double it." In taking the risk to disclose yourself, you confront directly your tendency to withdraw into your own world of brooding. Acting against your urge to do nothing, you gain a sense of control over your life, which can energize you.

The benefit of reaching out to others is contentment. The cost of staying isolated is loneliness.

RECEIVE ACCEPTANCE

Your depressed mind expects to be judged and rejected by others. After all, you see nothing of value in yourself and imagine others see you in the same way. You live in a trance of unworthiness, so you hold yourself back. Why place yourself in danger by letting people know you and exposing your faults? It only gives them ammunition for attacking you. However, others are not really the enemy who attacks you. You wage war against yourself. You measure yourself by impossible standards and constantly feel like a failure. Your inner critic, who focuses on the negative, keeps you down. It exaggerates your faults and minimizes your virtues, making you reluctant to share your inventory.

How can you free yourself from your fear of judgment and rejection? Telling another about your wrongdoing brings you face-to-face with your fear. It presents an opportunity to unmask it. Your humble, honest, courageous self-exposure inevitably invites a favorable response from your listener. Instead of the expected rejection, you receive an open-armed acceptance. The surprise may shock you into awareness that forgiveness is available for even the most grievous faults. As if by some miracle, feeling forgiven opens your heart to forgive yourself.

The benefit of risking rejection is surprising acceptance. The cost of holding back is remaining a slave to your inner critic.

EXPERIENCE HUMILITY

Scratch the surface of a pessimist and you find an idealist who is disappointed in himself and his life. In your depression, you become a well-practiced actor living out a tragic drama. Most often, you assume the role of a loser, a failure in life. What you hide are the grandiose expectations you have for yourself. You display the disappointment of not living up to them. Occasionally, you may put on the smiling face of success. You push yourself to look good and accomplish much. However, the momentary optimism disguises your lack of self-worth. Eventually, you crash, unable to sustain the façade.

A false sense of pride drives you to maintain some image that hides your true self. You take a major step toward humbly accepting yourself by admitting your faults to another. You come out of hiding behind the mask. You no longer have to be an actor in the drama of your life. What you risk in telling the truth about yourself is losing your pride and your shame. What a relief, giving up the burden of maintaining the pretense of a false self.

In reality, you are an ordinary human being, like everyone else, with strengths and weaknesses. Therein lies your true dignity. Simply being yourself means you have nothing to prove, nothing to defend, and nothing to live up to. As the *Tao Te Ching* puts it:

> **When you are content to be simply yourself**
> **And don't compare or compete,**
> **Everybody will respect you (8).**

Most importantly, you will respect yourself.

The benefit of risking humiliation is the letting go of your pride. The cost of not taking the chance is the relentless drive to continue proving how good you are.

CONFRONT SELF-DECEPTION

Drugged by your depressed mood, you are sedated and numb. Your mind is in a fog. You cannot think clearly, focus your attention, or remember what happened a few moments ago. You dwell an uncomfortable distance from yourself. In your depressed state of mind, you do not know what you want, what will make you happy, or how to behave. You feel only pain and senselessness.

When you take the fifth step, you invite another to bear witness to your sorrow and the suffering you cause yourself and others by your selfishness. You expose the pride, greed, anger, and other faults that underlie your mood. Furthermore, your honest self-disclosure also invites honest feedback from your listener. You gain another perspective on your behavior. Perhaps you exaggerated or minimized your faults, or did not look deeply enough into them. You may even ask your listener for advice and counsel, which can give you helpful direction on the perilous road of recovery. You do not have to travel alone. Taking the fifth step commits you to working with others on the path to healing and growth.

The benefit of letting another know you is the gift of honesty. The cost of keeping yourself hidden is a life of illusion.

SHOW YOUR STRENGTH

Your depressed mind focuses on what is missing, on scarcity, and on failures. Your mind runs on a single track, and its cargo is negativity. The final destination is despair. You disqualify anything positive in your life. You only see your weaknesses, shortcomings, and failings. No one can convince you that you have value as a person.

By admitting your weaknesses to another, you actually show your strengths. It takes honesty, humility, and courage to expose yourself. You can acknowledge your faults only after taking an honest look at yourself. Refusing to hide behind your façade of superiority or inferiority requires humility. Risking the judgment and rejection of another confronts your craving for approval. That takes courage. Displaying your strengths gives you and another person a glimpse of the personal goodness and abundance that lies behind your depressed face.

The benefit of admitting your weaknesses is appreciating your hidden strengths. The cost of secretly dwelling on your faults is self-hatred.

SENSE OF GOD'S PRESENCE

Depression drains you of hope and energy. Preoccupied with all your painful losses, you fully expect the deprivation to continue into the future. You see endings without beginnings, losses without gains. Your sense of dread robs you of the energy to create a more positive future. You firmly believe your efforts will be fruitless. So you give up. You feel helpless.

Relationships generate energy greater than the energy of each individual separately. That is precisely the reason alcoholics formed a fellowship for mutual healing. Exposing your weaknesses to another and experiencing their acceptance releases a hidden power. The interaction releases the power of love. As Freud observed, healing comes through the love expressed in a relationship with another. You experience an abundance that gives you hope for the future.

Imagine two individuals in a relationship as two intersecting circles. Part of each circle is separate, while another area is shared. The meeting of the two circles creates a third oblong shape. The shared area has a relational energy, created by the contribution of each individual. That energy is greater than the sum total of the energy of each individual. You experience, in heart-felt intimacy, a Power greater than yourself, which comes from you, but is beyond you. That Power is life-giving.

Those of a religious temperament experience it as a sacred presence. As Jesus teaches, "Where two or three are gathered in my name, I am in their midst." John, the beloved disciple, wrote, "God is love. Whoever lives in love lives in God and God in him."

The benefit of meeting with others is the opportunity to encounter a Power greater than yourself. The cost of staying alone is a magnified feeling of powerlessness.

YOUR DIALOGUE PARTNERS

Once committed to admitting your character defects to another, you must choose your dialogue partner. The fifth step suggests three: God, yourself, and another. The honest self-revelation renews those relationships. Furthermore, there is a wisdom to the order of these personal revelations that gradually deepens your awareness and acceptance of your faults.

If you believe in a personal God, you can pray to Him in your own words. Have a conversation with God, as with a friend, about your wrongdoings. God already knows your heart. There is nothing to hide from Him. You can be honest in admitting your failings and ask for His mercy. What is important in feeling free to admit your faults to God is your renewed confidence that He is all-loving and merciful, not harsh and judgmental. You already judge yourself harshly enough.

If you do not believe in a Supreme Being, admitting your faults to God makes no sense. However, you can still listen to the deep longings of your heart for an "other" to listen attentively, accept unconditionally, and forgive without limit. The yearnings come as a still quiet voice that is easily unheard in the loud noise of everyday life. Stillness and silence are required to hear the longing for an accepting "other."

When you honestly admit your shortcomings to yourself in plain words they become more real. You stand up before yourself and say, "These are my faults. I'm better than that." You take full responsibility for your thoughts, feelings, and behaviors, without identifying with them. You refuse to blame others or to make excuses. In taking responsibility, you walk the middle path between self-loathing for not being perfect and pretending you are already perfect. You are human.

This middle path of full conscious awareness places you on a path to accept, work with, and learn from faults. The attitude of acceptance that can lead to fruitful change is beautifully expressed in a poem by Rumi, a Sufi poet, entitled, "The Guest House" (1).

This being human is a guest house.
Every morning a new arrival.
A joy, a depression, a meanness,
Some momentary awareness comes
As an unexpected visitor.

Welcome and entertain them all!
Even if they're a crowd of sorrows,
Who violently sweep your house
Empty of its furniture.

Still, treat each guest honorably.
He may be clearing you out
For some new delight.

The dark thought, the shame, the malice.
Meet them at the door laughing,
And invite them in.

Be grateful for whoever comes,
Because each has been sent
As a guide from beyond.

ADMIT TO WHOM?

When you decide to speak with another, the question arises, "To whom should I make this confession?" Because of the sensitive nature of your self-revelation, you will look for an individual with qualities that would benefit you. Above all, you need a person with whom you can feel safe. That person must be trustworthy, someone you know will keep your secrets safe and not gossip about you. You also want your confidant to be open-minded and not judgmental, someone who will really listen to you. Avoid anyone who tells you that you are special or the greatest. Such comments only inflate your ego, increasing your pride and shame. What you need most is sincere, whole-hearted acceptance. You may also seek a wise, prudent person who can give you valuable feedback.

Where can you find such a person? You may look among the ranks of the professionals, a counselor, physician, or clergyman. Admittedly, not all professionals possess the qualities you want in the person who will listen to your confession. You must choose carefully and wisely. You may also consider a close friend or a spouse who may already be aware of your defects of character. Or you may choose a relative stranger from a support group who has impressed you with their trustworthiness, openness, and wisdom.

WHAT YOU ADMIT

When you meet with your dialogue partner, it is important that you not stay general and abstract in talking about your faults. You do not simply say, "I fail like everyone else." That is not true. You fail in your own unique way, according to your personality and life experience. The devil is in the details. Take the risk to reveal the unpleasant details, the exact nature of your wrongs, so that your partner can know you as a person.

You may start by telling the person you are depressed. That in itself is a difficult admission because of the stigma attached to mental illness. Next, let the person know what you are depressed about. Tell them the exact nature of the loss you are suffering: a relationship, a job, your health, the death of a loved one, and so forth. Then, the most difficult and healing part is to admit what you learned about yourself through your depression. Admit the faults, which you cling to so desperately, that make you so depressed.

For example, I met with one elderly man who had lost his wife three years before. He was discouraged because he still had severe bouts of depression. "I don't know why I can't move on with my life," he complained. We talked at length about their relationship and what he missed specifically with her gone. After many sessions, he admitted, "I never realized how dependent I was on her and how hard it is for me to stand on my own."

The following are several other examples of how honestly exploring the loss can help you understand yourself:

"The loss of my job made me aware of how much I crave status and approval from others."

"When I didn't get the promotion I wanted, I learned how angry I get when I don't get what I want."

"When I got depressed over someone else getting a raise, I became aware of how envious I get."

"When I failed that exam, I learned how addicted I am to success and the need to be perfect."

"When my boyfriend left me and I obsessed so much about him, I discovered that I'm addicted to love."

"The losses on the stock market showed me how greedy and materialistic I am."

"Feeling so overwhelmed at having a baby helped me see how self-centered and lazy I really am."

"Being so upset about not making the sale showed me how much I need to be in control."

PARADOX OF PERFECTION AND IMPERFECTION

Your depressed mood reveals your compulsion to be perfect. Measured against your own high standards, you see yourself as a miserable failure. Our society also promotes constant progress in striving toward perfection. It proclaims, "Become better every day." Hearing that message only makes you feel worse about yourself. You are stuck in your desire to be perfect and your hopelessness to attain it. You reject yourself as a flawed person.

Flaws, however, can hide beauty. There is a story about a famous artist. The city council of Florence purchased a six ton block of marble to create a monument for the city. They tried to commission the best sculptors in the city for the project. All refused, saying, "The marble is too imperfect. It will not be able to stand on its own." That huge block of marble sat in a field for 25 years. Then one day a young artist approached the council and said, "I'll make it into a masterpiece." When the huge block was delivered to his studio, the young man slept with it. Each night he hugged it and spoke to it, "What is crying out to be released from you?" After several weeks, he began his work. Two years later, he revealed his creation, which amazed the whole city. The statue was of David. The sculptor was Michelangelo.

Recovery presents you with a paradox in facing your flaws: "You are already perfect in your imperfection." As much as you hate your mood and your faults, your imperfections possess an unseen beauty. Look beneath the surface of your life. Look beyond and through your flaws. You were created perfect, with more goodness than you realize. Through understanding and accepting your weaknesses, you can release a magnificent beauty and power that is crying out to be acknowledged. Your unique beauty will be expressed through your imperfect, human personality.

PRACTICE: LOVING-KINDNESS

A traditional Eastern practice to uproot fear is called *metta*, or loving-kindness (2). According to legend, it originated when a group of frightened monks approached the Buddha for help. They were being sent into the forest to meditate, but their fear and sense of help-lessness stopped them. They heard stories about rampaging elephants, poisonous snakes, and ferocious tigers attacking people. As an antidote to their fear, the Buddha taught them the following practice of loving-kindness. It is noteworthy that he did not tell them to stay out of the forest or offer them physical protection. He approached their fear and dread as an affair of the mind and proposed a practice of mind training.

The practice is deceptively simple and powerful, engaging an unseen power within you:

1) Sit comfortably in a quiet place. Close your eyes and focus on the rhythm of your breath. Breathe deeply from your abdomen and allow the muscles of your body to relax. Sense the warmth of your breath radiating into your tense muscles, loosening the knots.

2) Once relaxed, consider for a moment where you are in life. Allow yourself to feel the stress, turmoil, and confusion. If you are preoccupied with your fault-finding expedition, feel deeply the guilt, shame, and disappointment in yourself.

3) Then select and focus your attention on phrases that address the pain and turmoil you feel in the moment. Express them as heart-felt wishes for yourself. For example, say to yourself: "May I be happy." "May I be free from sadness and sorrow." "May I feel content with my life." "May I be kind and loving." "May I be patient with myself." "May I forgive myself." Add whatever wishes best express your deepest desires in the moment.

4) Repeat three or four phrases to yourself for a period of time. Repeat the phrases slowly and thoughtfully for about ten minutes. Coordinate the repetition of the phrases with the rise and fall of your breath. Allow the words to sink into your mind and body.

This exercise fosters an attitude of loving-kindness toward yourself. It is the perfect antidote to fear and self-hatred. You can extend loving-kindness wishes to others in your life, radiating out towards your loved ones, towards anyone you encounter, towards those who harmed you, and towards the entire world.

It is a great risk to admit your faults to another. You may be rejected and feel worse about yourself. However, taking the risk sets you on a path to renew yourself and all your relationships. In humbling yourself, you let go of a false pride that only imprisons you in misery. You connect with yourself and others in a way that makes you feel alive.

11

Prepare the Way
A Humble Request

Step Six: "Were entirely ready to have God remove all these defects of character."

Step Seven: "Humbly asked Him (God) to remove our shortcomings."

"It is not I who create myself, rather I happen to myself."

—Carl Jung

"And as to me, I know of nothing else but miracles."

—Walt Whitman

While in the midst of the dark forest, a fierce wind begins to blow. The trees bend to the point of breaking. The branches and leaves brush against your face. The distant light remains your guide and keeps you moving forward despite your fear. The rushing wind through the trees moves the shadows about wildly, mixing with your shadow. They take grotesque shapes, like nocturnal ghosts. You feel completely engulfed by them, terrified for your safety. You cover your face in panic and cry out, "Help me! Please, someone help me!"

Steps six and seven work in tandem and deepen your humility. You come to recognize the power of your character defects to shape your life and your attachment to them. You further realize that you cannot help yourself. Only God can remove your faults. You do your part in becoming ready, and then surrender to let God do His part.

EATING HUMBLE PIE

Humility is a thread that runs through all the Steps. What is humility? You may think of it as being humiliated and put down. Already lacking self-esteem, you want to avoid that kind of humility. However, the root word of humility, "humus," gives a clue to its actual meaning. Humus means "earth," "ground." It is also the root word for "human." Being humble reminds us of the truth of who we really are as human beings. We come from the earth and return there. We share in all of material creation and live with our feet standing firmly on the ground.

Hooked on depression, your mind is lost in the clouds. You become preoccupied with how your life should have been and should be. Of course, your life never measures up to your grandiose expectations. You dwell on what is missing and become depressed. You lose your groundedness. A realistic sense of your relationships with yourself, others, and God (Universe) disappears.

Working the Steps humbles you gradually. Slowly, you come to an awareness and acceptance of the truth about yourself. You begin by admitting your powerlessness over your mood and the circumstances of your life. That can be a difficult admission, the result of many failures to find relief. Then, you must take an honest look at all the character defects that your depression hides. You imagined that your painful mood was your problem, but learned that it was only a symptom. Next, in the fifth step, you expose your faults to another and risk their judgment. You already judge yourself severely and imagine others are doing the same. Now, in the sixth and seventh Steps, you look more deeply at the roots of your character defects and ask for help. You willingly give up control and allow another to change you. Furthermore, and astoundingly, you are invited to lovingly embrace your weaknesses. All these Steps are a frontal assault on your pride.

What does it take to be humble? It takes experiences that bring you to your knees and open your heart to a new life. The Steps/Traditions book expresses this truth clearly: "For us, the process of gaining a new perspective was unbelievably painful. It was only by repeated humiliations that we were forced to learn something about humility. It was only at the end of a long road, marked by successive defeats and humiliations, and the final crushing of our self-sufficiency, that we began to feel humility as something more than a condition of groveling despair" (p. 72). Already feeling defeated by your depression, you may not be inclined to engage further in the humbling work of cleaning house.

NOT READY: THE BLAME GAME

Always realistic, the Steps/Traditions book admonishes: "Even then the best of us will discover to our dismay that there is always a sticking point, a point at which we say, 'No, I can't give this up yet.' And we shall often tread on even more dangerous ground when we cry, 'This I will never give up'" (p. 66).

What are your sticking points that make you hesitate to give up your faults and moods?

Anger, whether or not you acknowledge it, accompanies your depressed mood. Life has disappointed you in some way. You are angry at the losses you have endured. You use the anger stick against yourself, others, and God (or fate, the universe, or life). The name

Satan means "the accuser." In your compulsive blaming, you exercise demonic qualities that cut you off from the Source of happiness.

Troy, disappointed in himself:

"I'm trapped in a dead-end job. In fact, I work two jobs just to make ends meet. It's all my fault that I'm in this situation. I never cared about school and just goofed around. My parents and teachers tried to motivate me and warn me. But I ignored them. I smoked pot and hung around with the burn-outs. I dropped out of school in the tenth grade. My parents tolerated my doing nothing for only so long and made me get a job. I know I'm an intelligent person. I just wasted my abilities and never went to college. I know it does no good now, but I keep beating myself up for all my stupid mistakes."

The first target of your anger is yourself. You rehearse in your mind all your failures from the past. You keep a regret record in your mind. Regrets define your life. You continue to suffer the consequences of your poor decisions and feel sorry for yourself. You complain to others about your miserable lot in life. You continue to punish yourself for your sins with self-recriminations. "If only…" rules your life. Stuck in self-blame, you do not stop to consider what you can do now to improve your life.

Cynthia, mistrustful of others:

"I've been hurt so many times by coworkers, family, and supposed friends that I keep a journal of the insults I've suffered. When anyone hurts me, I don't allow myself to forget. So I write it down in my journal and keep myself on guard. 'Hurt me once, shame on you; hurt me twice, shame on me.' That is my motto. I read my journal regularly just to remind myself of the threat some people are to me. I won't allow them to harm me again."

The second target of your anger is others. You blame them for all your sorrow and pain. You may see yourself as a sensitive person who must protect yourself from the insensitivities of others. The world of relationships is, for you, a dangerous place. To survive, you must be cautious and alert. You collect your wounds and savor them. Preoccupied with blaming others, you neglect to look at yourself. You do not recognize how you hold grudges. You fail to see how the hostility and suspicion rob you of peace and others of your friendliness.

Marian, grieving her dead son:

"Our seven year old son died of cancer five years ago. He was the joy of my life. Not a day goes by that I don't think about him. I miss him so much. Our family and friends try to comfort me, but nothing seems to help. My grief is inconsolable. When I see parents with their children, I'm reminded that he's gone and break down in tears. It's not fair. I don't understand why God took him away. I will never be happy again."

A third target of your anger and grief may be God, Reality, Fate, or Life itself. Holding on to your grief, you accumulate grievances. You see life as cruel and depriving. The losses you suffer inevitably mount up and you cannot escape the pain. In reality, you focus your attention on the past and on what you have lost. Your world revolves around your pain. In addition, you may expect everyone else's worlds to center on your pain and demand their sympathy. Blaming God or the Universe, you make yourself a helpless victim.

HIDDEN BENEFITS

You may realize the uselessness of blaming. However, beyond useless, it is harmful. It reinforces your sense of helplessness, making you assume a victim role. Nevertheless, you feel powerless to stop it. But are you really powerless? Perhaps you hang on to the blaming because it benefits you in some way. It deflects responsibility from yourself. You then can avoid looking closely at yourself and taking responsibility for your own behavior.

Although you hate the discomfort of your depression, you may secretly love your condition. It works for you! That may come as a shock. Naturally, you want to get rid of the painful feelings. But character defects accompany your depressed reactions, and you are more reluctant to let those go. In fact, being depressed and withdrawing from life may provide unacknowledged benefits. The Steps/Tradition book realistically states: "What we must recognize now is that we exult in some of our defects. We really love them" (p. 66).

Loving your illness keeps you stuck. Victims have status.

BECOMING READY TO LET GO

What does it mean to be entirely ready? It means making a whole-hearted commitment to take decisive action. Of course, being entirely ready to let go of both your mood and faults does not occur all at once. It takes time and effort. The process involves digging deeper into your unconscious motivations for your behavior. Because much of your motivation is unconscious, you cannot easily know it. However, if you pay close attention to yourself you can discern signs of it operating. Specifically, your underlying motivation reveals itself in your self-image and in an analysis of the costs and benefits of your self-portrayal.

STORY TELLING: GHOSTS IN THE BASEMENT

Whenever I meet with patients, I invite them to tell me their stories. They tell me about what is bothering them and who they are. As the therapy progresses, their self-narratives unfold. Together we explore the meaning of their lives and the many ways they think about themselves. I tell them, "That's an interesting way to think about yourself. How did you learn to think that way?" We then explore childhood influences and consider alternative ways of thinking. The personal narratives of their lives shift as they gain understanding. Their simple black and white self-portraits become richer, more complex, and more colorful.

Your story reveals your underlying mood. In turn, your mood tells you about yourself. Examine it closely. What you are depressed about reveals your values and sensitivities. It shows what you love and hate. It is a window to your soul. Pay particular attention to the thoughts that arise when you are depressed. Notice also the persisting pattern of thoughts, which gather to shape your self-identity. This task may take some concerted effort because your mind may be sedated and foggy.

When I meet with my depressed patients, I always ask them, "What is making you depressed?" They may then report some events that went awry in their lives. I also ask them, "What goes through your mind when you are depressed?"

"I don't know. My mind is blank," they often say.

I then invite them to pay close attention to their thoughts and explain, "An emotional reaction lasts for only about ninety seconds. The uncomfortable physical sensation comes and goes quickly. What prolongs and intensifies it are the negative thoughts and the stories you tell yourself. You imagine catastrophic losses and dwell on your hopelessness and helplessness. Your mind creates commentaries about the situation."

The depressive thoughts are imbedded in stories you tell yourself. Why do you tell yourself such stories if they prolong the pain? The depressed mind feels distressed by change and the inevitable pain of endings. To create a sense of stability and security, you make commentaries about your life. You manufacture an image of yourself that gives you a sense of identity and purpose. These personal narratives become written in stone, fixed ideas that guide your self-understanding and behavior.

The story writing begins in early childhood when you can talk. Then you are able to put your experiences into words. That introduces a distance between your thinking and your immediate experience. Your personal stories are shaped by the messages you receive from your parents and from society beginning in early childhood. Their voices are ghost-like and godlike, roaming in your unconscious mind. They reflect your early emotional programming—how you learn to cope with life and find happiness. These childlike narratives become the lenses through which you view your experiences even as an adult. They are the scripts for the unfolding drama of your life.

You likely tell yourself, "I'm a depressed person." Labeling yourself as depressed organizes your complex experience of sadness. Captivated by significant loss, you feel helpless and hopeless. You view yourself as inadequate and worthless and see the world in pessimistic terms. Fatigue and a desire to withdraw from life possess you. Your assumed identity as a depressed person provides you with an explanation for your painful thoughts, feelings, and sensations. You may hang on to that label for dear life.

The following are three typical stories that you may tell yourself, being a victim, a loser, or a helpless child.

George, victimized by life:

"I was the youngest child. When I was born, my parents were old and tired. They didn't pay much attention to me, except to yell at me when I did something wrong. I did a lot wrong. I couldn't sit still and pay attention in school and had trouble getting my work done. The nuns yelled at me. They accused me of being lazy. They punished me and told my parents, who then punished me again. Everyone was against me. They told me I would never succeed in life. I believed them. I still do."

If you see yourself as a victim, you constantly tell yourself, "The world is a dangerous place; I can't protect myself." You live with a sense of helplessness in a threatening world. You are acutely sensitive to the dangers around you, always vigilant. You mistrust the motives of others, particularly those in authority who have power over you. Because you suffered terrible things in the past, you fear that the painful past will repeat itself in the future, so you are always on guard. Pessimism and doubt grip your mind. Caution rules your life. You manage your anxiety by being alert and seeking control, clarity, and certainty. However, fear poisons your quest for safety and security.

Arnold, a born loser:

"Kids teased me mercilessly when I was growing up because I was overweight. They called me 'Fatso' and 'Loser.' It didn't help that I had trouble in school. I never fit in with any group in high school. I was the outcast. I never succeeded at anything I did, so I gave up trying and spent a lot of time alone. I knew I wasn't going anywhere in life. I was too self-conscious to date and am still single. Now I have a lousy job making minimum wage. What kind of future can I look forward to?"

If you view yourself as a loser or a reject, you tell yourself, "I can't do anything right, and everybody knows it." Preoccupied with all your failures, you begin to become a collector of remembered defeats. As your failures accumulate over time, you create an identity for yourself as a loser. Others validate it in their rejection of you. In fact, their rejection matches your own. You firmly believe that you cannot succeed in life and give up making an effort. Your self-loathing and passivity lock you into self-defeating behavior.

Sophia, a helpless child:

"My parents spoiled me, and everyone called me 'the little princess.' I married a man who adored me and spoiled me like my parents did. When my husband died suddenly of a heart attack, I was completely lost. I keep his ashes in an urn on the fireplace so I can feel his closeness. I talk to him every night and tell him how much I miss him. My son tells me I haven't let go of his dad. He's right. I can't tolerate the idea of him being gone and me on my own."

Viewing yourself as a child, you say, "I'm helpless and need someone to take care of me." Your depression may drain you of energy and initiative. You feel helpless. "I can't" becomes your middle name. The more you withdraw from responsibilities in life, the more needy and helpless you feel. Your passivity and helplessness shout for others to take care of you. You come to believe that you cannot care for yourself. Feeling so dependent on others, you refuse to grow up. You become like Peter Pan.

DECONSTRUCTING THE STORY

When you pay close attention to your personal stories about yourself, you realize they are just stories. They are fiction created by your own imagination. You draw material from the many messages you received from childhood. Adults may have labeled you as self-centered, childish, lazy, inadequate, worthless, and so forth. Society said you must be rich, famous, popular, perfect, and so forth. These messages are ghosts in the basement of your unconscious mind. They make a lasting impression on the way you think about yourself.

Acknowledge that your self-image is composed of thoughts that come and go. It is not as solid or true as you think. T.S. Eliot, the word master, cautions against reliance on the truth of words: "Words strain, crack and sometimes break under the pressure, under the burden, under the tension, slip, slide, decay with imprecision, will not stay in place, will not stay still"(1). You alone give your ideas and words weight and truth. Perhaps you believe so much in that image because it gives you the illusion of security and stability in your topsy-turvy world. "This I know to be true about myself," you say. However, the label you give yourself, if taken literally, only imprisons you. It robs your freedom, keeping you from simply being yourself in the moment.

COST/BENEFIT ANALYSIS OF YOUR SELF-IMAGE

When my patients tell me their stories and label themselves, I ask, "What purpose do you think it could serve for you to think about yourself that way?" I invite them to engage in an analysis of the costs and benefits of their habitual way of thinking. I encourage them to involve their wise, rational mind in the work. With some reflection, you may be surprised to discover that you derive any benefit from labeling yourself. However, you also pay a severe price.

If you define yourself as a "depressed person," what are the possible benefits of thinking that way?

- You are justified to withdraw to take care of yourself, to adjust to the loss.

- You take time to re-evaluate your life and find new meaning in the loss.

- You discover and let go of your attachments.

- Others may offer sympathy and show compassion.

- You can learn compassion for others who are suffering.

But, what are the possible costs of this self-label?

- You disengage from your responsibilities.

- You dwell on the painful past and can become stuck.

- You identify with the sick role and expect others to care for you.

- You may continue to indulge in self-attacks.

- Your experiences validate your sense of worthlessness.

If you identify yourself with the "victim role," what are some advantages for you?

- You are acutely aware of your vulnerability and take steps to protect yourself.

- You are cautious in trusting and loyal when you find someone trustworthy.

- You can be confident and courageous in facing your fears.

- You are willing to fight for the underdog.

- Others may offer you sympathy and want to help.

But, what are some disadvantages of the victim role?

- You may indulge a sense of helplessness and not take action.

- You may blame others for your problems and not take responsibility.

- Others may try to exploit your weakness.

- Fear and doubt may rule your life.

- Always suspicious, you may isolate yourself for protection.

If you identify yourself as a "loser," what are the possible payoffs in assuming this role?

- You feel relieved from any responsibility to keep trying.

- Others feel sorry for you.

- You do not have to take risks to create a new life for yourself.

- You can feel safe and secure in doing nothing.

- You have a built-in excuse for poor performance.

But, what are some possible drawbacks in identifying yourself as a loser?

- You stay stuck with your sense of failure.

- Others may look down on you.

- You never experience the satisfaction of accomplishments.

- Your self-esteem remains low.

- Failure becomes a self-fulfilling prophecy.

If you see yourself as a "child," what do you gain?

- You do not have to take responsibility for yourself or others.

- You and others expect little from you.

- Others may want to take care of you.

- You can avoid the anxiety of growing up and facing new situations.

- You can remain innocent and naïve about evil in the world.

But, what do you lose in viewing yourself as a child?

- You never experience the satisfaction of taking on new challenges.

- Others may try to take over your life.

- You continue to feel needy and helpless, dependent on others.

- You lack courage to assert yourself and pursue your desires.

- You never grow up.

You develop your own life story as a way of making sense of the chaos of your experiences. These stories also reveal your habitual self-image, your sense of personal identity and your perceived strengths and weaknesses. They express your deep longings for safety, security, control over your life, affection, approval, and many other natural desires. Investigating these stories more deeply can help you appreciate the emotional investment you make in perceiving yourself the way you do. Withdrawing some of that emotional energy can free you to be yourself.

What makes you cling to your treasured personal narrative? It is fear. The fixed idea about who you are becomes a rock in the rushing river of life. You fear drowning in the rush of life, adjusting to so many uncontrollable changes. Standing on that rock, you feel safe and dry. But you are not swimming freely with the flow of your life. Fear rules and restricts your life. An AA saying reminds you, "Change only happens when the pain of holding on is greater than the fear of letting go."

"Perfect love casts out all fear" (I John 4:18). Turning to God in prayer, you open your heart to His love. The power of that love heals you.

PRAYER CHANGES YOU, NOT GOD

The seventh step invites you to pray to God. Why pray to Him? What does it accomplish? If you do not believe in a personal God, prayer makes no sense. It is having a conversation with nobody, with someone who does not exist. However, being still and meditating may put you in contact with a hidden Source of strength within.

Even if you do believe in God, how does it make sense? Why do you need to ask God for anything? God, who is all-knowing, already knows what you need. All-loving, He gives it to you. As Jesus says in the Sermon on the Mount (Matthew 6:32-33): "Your heavenly Father knows all that you need. Seek first his kingship over you, his way of holiness, and all these things will be given you besides." Nevertheless, Jesus also taught the power of prayer in the same sermon (Matthew 7:7): "Ask, and you will receive. Seek, and you will find. Knock, and it will be opened to you."

How can you make sense of such contradictory advice? The answer involves a deeper look at the nature of prayer. As a child, I was taught that prayer is a lifting up of the mind and heart to God. Now I consider it an opening of my mind and heart to God. It is more about listening than talking. It is more God's action than mine. That can be a humbling experience because it involves giving up control to God. The act of praying, of asking God specifically for something, transforms us. How does that happen?

Imagine you are attending a symphony. You go because you want something, the pleasure of listening to beautiful music. You consciously intend to be entertained. But as you become immersed in the music, you are captivated by its beauty and power. You are not conscious of the individual notes played or the instruments in the orchestra. You are caught up in the music. You lose yourself. For the moment, you are transformed. Totally absorbed in the present moment, you become the music. What an exhilarating experience that transcends your initial intention to be simply entertained. A Power greater than yourself possesses you.

Prayer may begin with a conscious intention. You want something from God and ask for it specifically. However, as you become more immersed in the act of praying, your faith is aroused. You sense God's presence in a new way, outside and within you. You experience, at a deep level, the power of His love and the tenderness of His concern. In the process, you lose yourself, that is, all your conscious striving. You acknowledge your powerlessness to change yourself through analyzing and working at your problems. Your self-centeredness begins to dissolve. Humility is born. Whatever you were asking for becomes less relevant because you sense you are being transformed through the praying. You become one with God. Your only desire is to do His will, "to seek first his kingship over you."

Prayer from the heart transforms your consciousness, giving you a new mind and heart with which to engage in your daily life. It releases the Higher Power that is both within and beyond you. It gives you hope in the midst of defeat while battling your demons.

TRANSFORM, NOT REMOVE

What do you pray for? You pray to remove your defects of character, as if they are dirt on the surface of your psyche that can be swept away without leaving a trace. However, your faults are more like deep stains that penetrate near the core of the person. They are deeply imbedded in your unconscious from birth and early childhood. Your faults represent misguided attempts to cope with the pain and emptiness of your life. They are attempts to fill the hole in the soul. You seek happiness, but look in the wrong place. In reality, your hated vices are distortions of your strengths, which need to be redirected to attain true happiness.

Consequently, the better strategy is to learn to transform, not remove, your shortcomings.

A traditional story illustrates the transforming strategy. Once upon a time, a poisoned tree grew in the middle of a village. All the elders gathered to decide what to do. One group saw only the danger in the tree's presence and recommended, "Let's cut it down before anyone is harmed." A second group countered, "Let's not hate it or fear it. After all, it's part of nature, which is good, and must be respected. We must have compassion for the tree because we share its nature. Let's build a fence around it so we will not get too close and get poisoned." The leader of the group listened to all the arguments and finally spoke up: "This poison tree is perfect, exactly what our village needs. Let's learn its secrets. Instead of destroying it or avoiding it, let's pick the poisoned fruit. Let's investigate it carefully and look for ways to use the poison as medicine to heal ourselves and others." Hearing that wisdom, all the elders stood up to affirm the decision.

The story suggests caution in trying to uproot your depression and underlying attachments too quickly. You may become impatient with yourself because your mood and faults persist despite your best efforts. Trying to eliminate them may be an act of violence against yourself which only intensifies your sadness and self-hatred. Remember your powerlessness over your mood. Learn the lesson of humility.

A more useful approach is to lean into your feelings and learn their message. Observe and investigate closely the stream of sensations, feelings, thoughts, and stories to uncover their hidden treasure. Be open to the possibility that the seeds of virtue have been planted in your vices.

A THORN IN THE FLESH

For example, in the Christian tradition, Saint Paul is known as a passionate man. He was a devout Jew who persecuted the early followers of Jesus because he saw them as heretics. After his sudden conversion, he became a staunch and irrepressible missionary for the Gospel. He travelled throughout the Mediterranean preaching, teaching, and writing about Jesus the Christ. Even as an apostle to the Gentiles, Paul remained a man of many passions, which were often in conflict within him. He confessed, "I cannot even understand my own actions. I do not do what I want to do but what I hate…What a wretched man I am!" (Romans 7:15, 22).

To resolve this painful inner conflict, Paul turned to prayer. He recounts, "…in order that I might not become conceited I was given a thorn in the flesh, an angel of Satan to beat me and keep me from getting proud. Three times I begged the Lord that this might leave me." His fervent prayer was answered in an unexpected way. "He said to me, 'My grace is enough for you, for in weakness power reaches perfection.' And so I willingly boast of my weaknesses instead…for when I am powerless, it is then that I am strong" (II Cor. 12:7-10). God did not remove the thorn in his flesh as he asked. Instead, through accepting his weaknesses, Paul learned humility and discovered a hidden power within.

PARADOX OF DOING AND NOT DOING

When I was a child learning to pray, I was taught: "Work as if everything depends on you; pray as if everything depends on God." My teachers were aware of the danger in ignoring either side of the equation of effort and grace. If we believe that only our efforts count, we can become arrogant with success or despairing with defeat. If we believe that God does it all, we can become passive spectators to our lives. Prayer prepares us for action, giving us confidence and direction. In turn, action, struggling to make a better life, brings us humbly to prayer.

The fellowship of Alcoholics Anonymous echoes this paradoxical wisdom, encouraging its members both to work the program and surrender to their Higher Power. It is not simply a self-help program. A cry for help is required. For example, the *Tao Te Ching* advocates both doing and not doing, letting events unfold naturally:

Less and less do you need to force things,
until finally you arrive at non-action.
When nothing is done,
nothing is left undone.
True mastery can be gained
by letting things go their own way.

It can't be gained by interfering (48).

Recovery from depression is like planting a garden and watching the flowers grow. It requires much effort to prepare the garden for growth. You cannot force flowers to bloom. They will not flourish unless you prepare the ground. You have to till the soil, plant the proper seeds, and pull weeds. Then the sun, rain, and warmth allow the seeds to sprout and show forth their natural beauty. The hidden power of nature works its wonders. You watch and wait, tending the garden as needed, and witness the miracle of new life.

In the same way, you cultivate the garden of your soul. You remove the weeds of your shortcomings and plant seeds of good works. Prayer, meditation, and spiritual practices nurture the plants. You work at removing any obstacles that interfere with the emergence of your true self, which is naturally good, wise, and sane. The gift of new life cannot be suppressed if the mind and heart are open and willing.

PRACTICE: WRITE YOUR LIFE STORY

We all have a unique story to tell. We live our lives day after day and create commentaries to explain our experience to ourselves and others. Our experience can be confusing and baffling. We create personal narratives to give meaning to our lives and to connect with others. Intimacy grows in the exchange of our stories, through which we share ourselves.

Take a moment to reflect on your life and how it is unfolding. Begin at the beginning to understand what has influenced the way you are now. What were your parents like? How would you describe them? What qualities did you love and hate about them? What was their marriage like, and how did they parent you? What did you receive from them? Review in your mind all the significant people in your life, your siblings, relatives, and teachers. Notice their qualities, how they interacted with you. What messages did you receive from them? What did you receive from them? Gain a sense of their impact on your life.

Next, look at the important events in your life, the turning points. Some events were beyond your control, while others resulted from choices you made. Were there life-changing events, such as the death of a parent, physical or mental illness, or the birth of your children? What were the losses you suffered? How did you cope? When did your depressed mood first appear? How did you progress through school, your career, and your relationships? What important decisions did you make that changed the course of your life regarding marriage, children, and career? How did you make those decisions? Did you carefully evaluate the costs and benefits, react impulsively, or choose intuitively?

Stand back and observe the flow of your life, with all its fits and starts. What patterns do you notice, particularly in your shifting moods? What seems to be the trajectory, the direction, of your life? What seem to be the driving forces within and outside you? You can begin to understand your hidden motivations, your desires for security, power, or prestige. What were your passions and priorities?

Write your own autobiography. Be an astute observer of yourself, as if you were an historian investigating the life of an important person. Paint a collage of your life with the various events. I suggest you write an outline of significant events. If you are so inclined, expand that outline into a brief autobiography. You will notice that you have always been telling yourself stories about yourself, and these stories have changed over the years. Your self-conscious thoughts are not as solid and fixed as you think. You are also infinitely more than your thoughts about yourself, which cannot fully express your mystery.

Painful memories and confusing messages from your childhood may arise during this reflection. If you feel too overwhelmed by them, do not proceed. Some early life trauma may be coming to the surface and require you to talk with a professional. However, if you feel some sadness, stay with the feeling and memories. Explore the memories and messages to help you understand the influences that shaped the way you view yourself. Remember, your self-image is just another passing thought. It is not who you are as a person. You do not have to make it the ultimate guide of your life.

Uncovering your character defects in these steps launches you on a further search. Hopefully, nonjudgmental curiosity will move you to explore more deeply. Then you will be transformed by discovering the buried gold of virtue within your weaknesses and taking positive action.

Dennis Ortman, Ph.D.

12

Feeling Remorse
Forgiveness from the Heart

*Step Eight: "Made a list of all the persons we had harmed,
and became willing to make amends to them all."*

*Step Nine: "Made direct amends to such people whenever possible,
except when to do so would injure them or others."*

*"To exist is to change, to change is to mature,
to mature is to go on creating oneself endlessly."*

—Henri Bergson

"Boldness has genius, power, and magic in it."

—W.H. Murray

The light around you brightens. You move faster with confidence. You see more clearly the holes, rocks, and fallen branches on the winding path. Your heart quickens. Shadows still surround you, but they are less frightening. Then, you notice something new you never saw before. Along the path are colorful flowers. In the half-light you can see their beauty, their splendid variety of shapes and colors. You wonder if there are more wonders yet to be revealed in the brightening light. A desire arises in you and you exclaim, "I want to be in the light!"

"Steps Eight and Nine are concerned with personal relationships," the Steps/Traditions book (p.77) reminds us. There are two moments in taking these steps. First, you recognize the harm your attachment to depression causes you and others. Then, you take bold action to repair the damage and renew relationships. You commit to pursuing a vital, value-chosen life. The focus shifts from an inward look at your character defects and their roots to a backward and outward glance that leads to decisive action. Your efforts to clean house naturally overflow into helping others.

STUCK IN PAIN AND THE PAST

Caught up in depression, looking backward and outward and taking reparative action is tricky. Your tendencies toward preoccupation with your pain, getting lost in the past, and excessive self-blame interfere.

Katelyn, preoccupied with her health:

"I was diagnosed with irritable bowel syndrome and Crohn's Disease as a teenager. My stomach was a mess. It was so depressing. When I had attacks, I was in such pain that I could do nothing but lay in bed. I cried constantly and begged for relief. I could not tolerate any stress. An attack would surely follow. I was recently diagnosed with fibromyalgia and experience pain almost all the time. I feel like a cripple. Pain medications made me groggy. I just wanted to sleep. I got my medical marijuana card. Now I smoke every day just to cope with my life."

You may become absorbed by your emotional and physical pain. It is constantly on your mind. Your only thought is how to cope with it. Pain becomes the center of your life, and all your thoughts and activities revolve around the pursuit of relief. You may expect that others' worlds should also revolve around your pain, expecting sympathy and accommodation. When you are caught up in your pain, nothing else matters. You shun responsibilities and withdraw from life. You are unable to look outward to see the impact of your behavior on other people.

Randy, hanging on to grief:

"My father died fifteen years ago. He was a monster when we were growing up. He drank every day, had a terrible temper, and beat us. I never mourned his death. I was so angry with him that I refused to attend his funeral, even though my mother pleaded with me. Frankly, I was relieved that that SOB was dead. I became an angry and bitter man with an explosive temper. Through therapy after my divorce, I realized that I kept my father alive by becoming like him. The man I hated most, I imitated. A bond of anger kept us together. I never really let him go."

Unresolved grief can keep you a prisoner of the past. You cycle through stages of denial, depression, anger, and bargaining, but never come to acceptance of the loss. Not only do you mourn the loss of loved ones, but you grieve the loss of your fantasy of what life should have been. You may miss having the perfect parent or spouse and refuse to give up the shattered dream. You may unconsciously keep that person alive by identifying with their behavior, becoming like them in some way. Your preoccupation with the past interferes with your ability to assess realistically your own behavior.

Norma, obsessed with self-blame:

"I hate the holidays. The kids are excited about Santa Claus and all the gifts. I just go through the motions like a zombie, decorating, shopping, wrapping presents, and cooking. I feel like Scrooge, but I can't help it. I'm so depressed but don't know why. I have some vague sense that I'm inadequate and not doing a good enough job. My family compliments me and tries to lift my spirits, but it only makes me feel worse. I have no idea what I expect of myself. I simply feel the presence of a dark judge who keeps telling me I'm not measuring up."

You inner critic, the Judge, may never rest. She follows you like a black shadow you cannot escape. The faster you run, the harder you try, she is still there. Her voice continually berates you, saying that you are not performing well enough. Whatever you do is deficient. You may not even know the standards by which you are being judged. But you sense you can never measure up. The relentless negative judgments make you believe that you are defective as a person. In the critic's blaming shadow, you cannot fairly judge yourself.

The seventh step asks you to make a list of all the persons you have harmed. To make that list you need an expanded consciousness and an awareness of how you are part of a larger whole.

INTERCONNECTED

A traditional Jewish tale speaks about our interconnectedness. An old rabbi asked his students, "How can you tell when the night has ended and the day has begun?" Traditionally, that is the time for certain holy prayers. One student responded, "It is when you can see an animal in the distance and tell whether it is a sheep or a dog." The rabbi shook his head. Another student proposed, "It is when you can clearly see the lines on your hand." Again, the rabbi said, "No." A third student said, "It is when you can look at a tree in the distance and tell if it is a fig or a pear tree." "No," the rabbi answered. "Then, what is it?" the confused pupils asked. "It is when you can look on the face of any man or woman and see that they are your brother or sister. Until then, it is still night."

We are all members of the same human family. We have a single origin and share a common destiny. We all long for happiness and seek relief from suffering. More intimately, as Saint Paul suggests, we are members of one body. When one member suffers, all suffer. We are not as separate as we think.

Living in the information age, with instantaneous worldwide communication, we are more aware that we live together in a global village. The suffering of those across the world, from natural disasters, political unrest, or killing plagues, are brought into our living rooms. Their suffering calls out for our compassionate response. We see the impact of our political, economic, and environmental decisions reverberate across the planet. The divisions of national boundaries, race, and religion appear artificial. We share a common humanity, destiny, and responsibility to maintain our planet. We are not as separate as we think.

Our essential connectedness is stated clearly in the golden rule, to which all the religious traditions subscribe: "Treat others the way you would have them treat you" (Matthew 7:12). The love commandment echoes this truth: "You shall love your neighbor as yourself" (Matthew 22:39). That means loving your neighbor as another self. There is an inseparable link between how we treat others and how we relate to ourselves. In caring genuinely for others, we care for ourselves; in loving ourselves, we love others. The opposite also holds true regarding hatred and judgment: "If you want to avoid judgment, stop passing judgment...The measure with which you measure will be used to measure you" (Matthew 7:1-2). The hostility and judgment we impose on others boomerangs back to us.

We imagine making life-long choices between independence and dependence. The deeper truth is that we are interdependent, mutually dependent on each other. As we are becoming more aware of the current ecological crisis, interdependence extends beyond the realm of personal relationships to include the entire planet. The minerals, plants, and animals are also our brothers and sisters. The fate of the natural world determines our destiny as a human race. Our actions shape the future of the universe.

TAKE A LOOK, MAKE A LIST

What harm have you caused? The Steps/Traditions book states: "To define 'harm' in a practical way, we might call it the result of instincts in collision, which cause physical, mental, emotional, or spiritual damage to people" (p. 80). Aware of your responsibility for your own and others' wellbeing, step eight invites you to look honestly at how you have harmed yourself and others by indulging in your depressed mood.

SELF-HARM

Emotions Anonymous states clearly that before you can make amends with others you must acknowledge your own woundedness and need for healing: "Many of us realize the person hurt the most has been ourself, and we have to include our own name on the list" (p. 66).

After taking your moral inventory in step four, you realize that your depression is not the real problem, only a symptom of a deeper problem. Your depressed mood, as painful as it is, does not cause you real lasting damage. The feeling is distressful, but not dangerous. The real harm comes from the misguided ways you try to cope with your moods and from the distorted desires that give rise to the depression.

Your depressed mood signals that something is missing in your life, that you have gone off track. Instead of entering the heart of darkness to explore its meaning and learn its message, you may manufacture ways of avoiding and trying to control the pain. It is important that you recognize your own avoidance strategies. They are self-defeating and only cause you more harm. Some common misguided coping strategies are to drown yourself in activities as a distraction. That only leads to burnout. You may try to comfort yourself with some excessive indulgences, like overeating, shopping, sex, or gambling. A common way of self-medicating is to abuse alcohol or drugs. Their use may cover the pain briefly. However, inevitably, they will make you more miserable. A host of other problems follow in the wake of addictions.

Your depressed mood reveals both your losses and your longings. Remember that the word depression means "pressed down." Some life force within you is being suppressed and is calling out for attention. You only have to listen closely and then act. Your sense of loss shows what you treasure that has been taken away from you. Your mood invites you to withdraw from your normal occupations to explore what is missing. In your fourth step work, you may have discovered your craving for love, approval, power, accomplishment, security, or perfection. You looked at your inflated expectations and your false belief that satisfying these desires would make you happy. Pursuing these excessive desires only brings suffering.

Your mood disguises your deep longings for wholeness and aliveness. These yearnings come from your true self, which is basically good, brave, and sane.

Depression, feeling dead inside, is a protest against the suppression of these energizing desires. Your depressed mind of dissatisfaction focuses on what is missing in your life and ignores the potential for growth in suffering losses. It overlooks the abundance that surrounds you. However, the gift of tears enables you to let go of the pain of loss and learn compassion. Your depression invites you to find meaning in your losses and discover what you value most. It also encourages you to recognize the many ways you have not cared for your physical, mental, emotional, and spiritual wellbeing.

Brittany, suffering post-partum depression:

"After my baby was born I became depressed. The birth was the happiest day of my life. I couldn't understand why I became so depressed. The doctor told me it was post-partum depression. I lost all interest in life and just wanted to sleep. I didn't even care about my baby, which shocked me. Fortunately, my mother stayed with us and cared for us. After a while, the guilt of not caring for my baby became overwhelming. I had a good talk with myself and reminded myself of how much I loved my child. I decided to push myself and gradually worked out of the depression."

OTHER-HARM

Alcoholics Anonymous is unflinching about the need for alcoholics to take this step for a genuine recovery: "Every AA has found that he can make little headway in this new adventure of living until he first backtracks and really makes an accurate and unsparing survey of the human wreckage he has left in his wake" (Steps/Traditions, p. 77). You may acknowledge that your depressed reactions have strained relationships, but may object that it has caused wreckage. You can see how it has ruined your life in many ways, robbing you of happiness. How has it damaged others' lives?

Your depression makes you withdraw within yourself. The harm you cause others may be more from what you fail to do in relationships than from what you do. You commit more sins of omission than commission. One patient, struggling to motivate himself, said, "The opposite of depression is ambition." Not surprisingly, those who love and care about you have been more deeply affected. Review your life and think about those you harmed, intentionally or not, by your depressed mood and behavior. Who are they? Consider the following observations and questions:

- When you are depressed you lose motivation and energy to be involved in life. What responsibilities did you neglect? How did it affect the persons who counted on you?

- You can become self-absorbed and act as if the world revolves around your pain. Did you lack empathy for the suffering of those close to you during your episodes? Did you become demanding of care from them?

- Because of all the losses you suffered, you may come to view yourself as a victim. Did you blame others for your misery? Did you feel sorry for yourself?

- Lacking self-confidence, you fear failing and confirming your sense of worthlessness. Did you avoid taking initiative at home or work, expecting others to pick up the slack?

- Depression has been described as anger turned inward. How did you express your anger? Did you become passive-aggressive with others, stubborn and withholding?

- During times of hopelessness and despair, have you attempted or threatened suicide? What was the impact on those who love you?

- When you felt hopeless and helpless, did you manipulate others to care for you or assume your responsibilities?

- Your sense of worthlessness results from your inflated expectations about yourself. Did you have similar unrealistic expectations of others? How did you show your disappointment in them? How did you react to their constructive criticism?

- Focusing on what is missing in your life you may become jealous of others. How did you express your envy? Did you demean others to build yourself up?

- You may feel desperate for love and approval. How manipulative or demanding were you for reassurance from others?

- Your pessimistic thinking may lead you to complain frequently. How did your complaining affect others? Were you pleasant to be around?

- Feeling powerless over your life, did you try to be controlling of others and your environment?

- Feeling insecure about yourself, you may put on a mask. You may try to create an image of yourself that others will like. How did living this lie affect others?

When two depressed people get together, they may unintentionally worsen each other's moods.

Diana, having marital conflicts:

"Both my husband and I are depressed. When I'm down, I withdraw and don't want to talk with anyone. My husband asks constantly, 'What's the matter? Did I upset

you? Did I do something wrong?' I try to reassure him that he did nothing to upset me, that I'm just in a bad mood. But he doesn't believe me. He continues to nag me with his questioning. Then, I really do get mad at him, yell, and feel worse. He feels worse too."

One by one, hold in your memory those you harmed. Recall the circumstances, the repeating situations, in which you caused that person pain. Bring to mind what you were experiencing during those incidents, your anxiety, your sense of desperation, and your selfish pursuit of relief. Put yourself in the place of the person you hurt and feel their pain. What did they experience? Imagine what they were thinking and feeling at the time. How were your actions harmful to them?

Be gentle with yourself during these recollections. Avoid blaming yourself or refusing any responsibility. Allow yourself to feel genuine remorse, which opens your heart in compassion. Such compassion is the only way to escape the prison of self-absorbing depression.

WILLING, NOT WILLFUL

In taking this step to make amends, you affirm your freedom. Your instincts cry out for certainty, clarity, and control. When you say you are willing to make amends, you take an active leap into the unknown. You take responsibility for your life and proclaim, "I fully accept the task to create a new life." The ultimate destination of growing maturity remains unknown, but you commit to the path nonetheless. You willingly leave behind the familiar prison of your depressed mood.

Do not underestimate the magnitude of this step, from contemplating harm done to repairing the damage. It is a weighty decision, like getting engaged to a loved one. Consider carefully the cost of staying passive in your depression, your unlived life. Believing in a Power greater than yourself, imagine the benefits of a life directed by what is important to you. For this new phase of your journey, you will need determination, boldness, and courage.

I ask my depressed patients, "What would you do if you weren't depressed?" They usually respond that they would socialize more, work harder, exercise more, spend more time with the family, and so forth. "What keeps you from doing those things?" I ask. "My depression does," they say. "Why do you give your mood so much power over your life?" "There's nothing I can do about it. I feel so helpless," they respond. In all honesty, you cannot hide behind your depression. You still have a choice.

You have already taken leaps of faith in admitting your powerlessness, in deciding to believe in a Higher Power, and in having God remove your faults. How do you gain the courage to make this new intentional leap? The AA saying reminds you, "Change only happens when the pain of holding on is greater than the fear of letting go."

An exercise recommended by psychologist Steven Hayes (1) can help you appreciate what is involved in making this decision. It can assist you in clarifying your values and what you are sacrificing in being stuck in depression. How do you want to live? According to the dictates of your mood or your chosen values?

Take a piece of paper and write down in order on the left hand side the following ten domains that might be important to you:

1. Marriage/couple/intimate relationship—being a loving partner.

2. Parenting—being a nurturing parent.

3. Family relations—supporting your larger family.

4. Friendship/social relations—being a reliable friend.

5. Career/employment—developing your talents.

6. Education/training/personal growth and development—growing as a person.

7. Recreation/leisure—enjoying life.

8. Spirituality—connecting with your Spirit.

9. Citizenship—contributing to society.

10. Health/physical wellbeing—staying healthy.

Perform this exercise in four steps:

1. Consider for a moment each of these areas and how important they are to you. Then, rank them in order of importance from 1 to 10. Write that number next to the domain.

2. Next, consider each area and ask yourself how important it is to you right now on a scale of 1 to 10, with 1 meaning not important at all and 10 meaning extremely valued. Write your responses in a column to the right of each area. Label that column "importance."

3. Thirdly, rate each area according to your current behavior. How well have you been living this value on a scale of 1 to 10? Write your response in another column to the right of the previous one. Label that column "actual behavior."

4. Finally, subtract the score of your actual current behavior from the importance score. Write the difference in a third column, labeled "gap," to the right of the last two. Notice the deviation between what you value and how you live. The size of the deviation represents how much you need to change to live a value-directed life.

What you are deciding in step eight is your willingness to work at narrowing the gap between what you value and how you are currently living. You know the pain of being trapped in your depression. Now you confront your fear of making a change.

TAKE BOLD ACTION: THE FORCE AWAKENS

The ninth step invites you to take action by making amends. How do you make amends? How do you repair the damage your mood caused you and others? *Emotions Anonymous* clearly states a two-step process beginning with yourself, "We must accept and forgive ourselves if we are to accept and forgive others" (p. 66).

MAKE PEACE WITH YOURSELF: SELF-COMPASSION

Acknowledging the harm your addiction to depression has caused can awaken in you compassion for your suffering. Your compassion, in turn, motivates you to make the commitment to care for yourself. Your mood causes physical, mental, emotional, and spiritual damage. Each area needs to be addressed in your recovery.

First of all, your depression drains you of energy and interest in life. You want to sleep, lose your appetite, and withdraw from your normal activities. Self-care requires you to act against the inertia of your mood. You need to push yourself to exercise, eat a proper diet, and establish a sleep schedule. Taking medications can assist in elevating your mood and energy level.

Secondly, a mind of dissatisfaction governs your thinking. Your thoughts run in one direction, toward the negative. You focus on what is missing in your life. Compared to the grandiose expectations you entertain, your life does not measure up. You reject yourself for being imperfect. The emotional result is sadness, disappointment, and discouragement.

How can you rebalance your thinking? You can consciously change the focus of your attention from what is missing to what you already have, from a preoccupation with scarcity to abundance. Be aware of the gravitational pull of your mind towards the negative. Stand firm as an observer with your spacious mind of abundance. You can embrace your wholeness, which includes your flaws. This perspective shift will fill your heart with gratitude, generosity, and hope.

Think of those who benefited you. Let your imagination transport you back through your life, beginning with your childhood. Think of those who showed you love, attention, and affection. Let the important people in your life come to mind: your parents, grandparents, aunts and uncles, relatives, friends, teachers, work associates. Hold each of these individuals for a few moments in your mind, one by one, and recall what they did to enrich your life. Allow your heart to fill with gratitude for their generosity and love. Whether these persons are living or deceased does not matter. They are still alive through you, in memory and in the ways they shaped your life.

Then take a few moments to express a heartfelt thanks to them, each individually. That is a way to make amends. Recall what you appreciated most about them and thank them for it. If that person is still alive, consider how you might express your gratitude to them personally. Expressing appreciation is just as important as apologizing when building relationships. Gratitude for being loved releases the power within you to transform your shortcomings into virtues. Love inspires love.

Thirdly, address harmful feelings. If you are depressed, you grieve many losses. Life itself and people have disappointed you. Your mind tends to focus on those who harmed you. You may even become a wound collector. Your sadness is mixed with anger at the unfairness of how you have been treated. While the anger may protect you, it also harms you. As the AA slogan states: "Having a resentment is like drinking poison and expecting someone else to die." Your anger consumes you. It deepens your sense of guilt and worthlessness. It clouds your clear vision of yourself and others. For healing, follow your resentment. Notice when it raises its ugly head. It cries out to be let go.

Gary, holding a grudge against his parents:

"Both my parents are alcoholics. My father beat me when he was drunk, and mother just stood by and did nothing. I left home as soon as I could. I haven't talked with my parents in years and have no interest in contacting them. They are getting older now. My friends tell me I'll regret not seeing them before they die. But I really don't care. I keep wondering what my life would be like if I was raised by loving parents instead of them."

The blaming holds you prisoner. Forgiveness frees you from the scourge of anger, hatred, and resentment. You forgive others for your own sake, to give you relief. Again, take a walk through your past, beginning with childhood. This time, recall those who harmed you and caused you suffering. This may be a painful walk, but take it with the confidence you gained from the memories of those who loved and supported you. Look honestly at your grudge list. One by one, hold in memory each of those persons who caused you pain. Hold them gently. Recall the painful incidents and how the person offended you. Allow yourself to feel the pain and your anger. Watch the hurt, sad, and angry emotions arise and fall away.

In your mind, tell the person how their behavior affected you, how it influenced your life. Imagine what you would say. Then put yourself in the place of that person. Try to imagine what that person was feeling, thinking, and doing when they harmed you. What motivated their actions against you? Did they realize they were hurting you? Imagine that person listening attentively to you as you express the suffering they caused you. Imagine also what that person would say to you now, aware of your suffering. You may want to write a letter to that person to express more clearly your feelings. You do not have to mail that letter.

Be gentle with yourself as you recall painful incidents in your life. Especially if you were traumatized by physical or sexual abuse as a child, you must be careful in remembering the past. The recollections may be too painful, too overwhelming, and cause flashbacks. If you begin to feel overwhelmed, stop immediately, take a deep breath, and try to calm yourself. Address the painful memories only when you feel strong enough and ready. Be gentle with yourself.

Finally, you can heal the spiritual damage, the despair and hopelessness, by entering into the heart of the darkness. Depression invites you to be silent and contemplate your life. Explore the meaning of your mood. Listen to the deep longings for wholeness. Reorient your life in the direction of your true values. In this process of repair, you will awaken the Life Force, the Power greater than your small self.

ASKING FORGIVENESS

Contrary to the sentimentalism of "Love Story," mature love means saying you are sorry when you have wronged someone. How can you make an apology from the heart?

First, you need to recognize honestly the impact of your mood-driven behavior on others. This requires empathy, the ability to step out of yourself and into the shoes of another. That may not be so easy for you because of your instinctive self-preoccupation with your own pain. Working step eight prepared you for making a sincere apology.

Secondly, seek forgiveness only when you are ready. It is an intimate act of exposing yourself that may arouse an overwhelming anxiety. Anticipate your fears in approaching each person on your list and how you can keep yourself calm enough to speak from your heart. Of course, you must be sincerely sorry for what you have done. Otherwise, your deceit will only cause more harm.

Thirdly, asking for forgiveness should be done face-to-face, not over the phone, text, or email. If you cannot meet with that person because of practical difficulties, you may decide to write a letter. One of my patients told me how she reconnected with an estranged friend by mail and felt immense relief. If the person is deceased or unavailable, you may hold that person in your mind, make a sincere apology, and pray for him or her.

Fourthly, make your apology specific, not general. Do not say, "Forgive me for whatever I may have done to hurt you." Before the meeting, have a clear idea of specific incidents, behaviors, or neglect that harmed that person. Do not make excuses for yourself. Do not use your depression as a justification for your hurtful behavior. Speak simply, directly, and honestly from your heart, as best you can.

Fifthly, allow the hurt party to respond, and then listen. Resist the urge to become defensive if that person becomes critical of you. Your inner critic may be easily activated by any angry response. Most likely, the offended person will be surprised and grateful for your apology and quickly accept it. That person may even try to take some of the blame and ask for your forgiveness. Be open to whatever happens. Do not become fixated on a particular outcome, as is your habit. Let it be an intimate moment.

Finally, realize that asking for forgiveness is just one step in the process of healing. Have a firm purpose of amending your own life, so that you will not harm that person or anyone else again. Keep pursuing your values. Of course, you will not succeed one hundred percent. Recovery is a work in progress, not perfection. Commit yourself to transform your vices into virtues. Learn from your inevitable relapses, allowing them to strengthen you.

WHAT TO TELL

Some may ask, "Should I tell the person about my depression?" You may wonder if that person will think you are making an excuse for yourself. You may also still feel shame about your condition and want to keep it secret. I advise that you decide for yourself. You have the right to privacy regarding your mental health condition. You also have the right to respect your sensitivity about being misunderstood and judged by others. Many, ignorant about mental illness, entertain prejudiced ideas about it. When you become secure within yourself about your condition, you may choose to tell others. Your honest and straight-forward speaking about it may help overcome the prejudiced thinking of many in our society.

Alcoholics Anonymous recommends caution in making amends: "Good judgment, a careful sense of timing, courage, and prudence—these are the qualities we shall need when we take step nine" (2). You need to consider whether your apology would really be beneficial for the person hearing it. Some cases can be complex and sensitive, such as revealing an infidelity. Consulting with a trusted friend or professional may be advisable in these circumstances.

Roger, feeling guilty for cheating:

"I had a one night stand on a business trip five years ago. I was feeling lonely, got drunk, and slept with a stranger I met in the bar. I feel terrible about it, so depressed. Not a day goes by that I don't suffer guilt pangs. I never told my wife. What good would it do? She would be so hurt and might even want a divorce. I keep wondering whether or not I should tell her to be honest and relieve my guilt. I love her and know I would never do it again."

PARADOX OF ACCEPTANCE AND CHANGE

Hooked on depression, you are discouraged. Life does not measure up to all your hopes. Even though you try mightily to improve yourself, you fail miserably. The harder you try, the worse you feel. Your mood worsens with each repeated failure to overcome your depression. You feel more helpless and hopeless.

Perhaps you are trying too hard and just need to relax with your condition. Then you discover a surprising paradox: "When I accept myself just as I am, I can change." Accepting your powerlessness to change your condition opens your heart and mind to grace. Paul Tillich, the noted theologian, defines grace: "Accept the fact that you are accepted, despite the fact that you are unacceptable." You refuse to accept so much because life does not conform to your high expectations. Letting go of your fixed ideas about what should have been and what should be can set you free. You are free to embrace your life as it is and be your true self.

Accepting your reality, with all its complexity, releases a hidden power that enables you to fulfill your true potential. Beneath the surface of your flawed existence resides a basic goodness, a sharing in Divine Life. You are good to the core. God does not make junk. Your depression tricks you into thinking you are worthless and must prove yourself. Simply let your goodness show by letting your natural virtues shine.

PRACTICE: TONGLEN

Your depression makes you want to withdraw from life to nurse your wounds. Grief, for a time, is natural and healing. However, when the mood becomes like a drug, you try to numb yourself to the pain and avoid life. Opening yourself to life and to others inevitably involves pain. If you allow yourself to care, you will hurt. Growth involves embracing and learning from your suffering. In the process, you develop courage and compassion.

A traditional Eastern practice to cultivate fearlessness and empathy is "Tonglen," which means "sending and receiving" (3). It counters your natural instinct to flee what is uncomfortable and chase after pleasure. Through this exercise, you receive with openness and compassion your own and others' suffering. Then you send out love and peace. Here are the steps in the practice:

1)   Sit comfortably in a quiet place with your eyes closed. Focus on the rising and falling of your breath. Breathe slowly and deeply, sensing peace and relaxation filling your body. With each breath, feel a sense of openness and spaciousness within your heart.

2)   Next, still focusing on your breath, imagine that you are breathing in hot, black, dirty smoke that repulses you. Feel your repugnance as you breathe in the burning blackness. As you breathe out, imagine you are exhaling a cool, gentle, fresh breeze that fills the room. Imagine the bright freshness of the great outdoors coming from within you. Breathe in tarry smoke and breathe out fresh air.

3)   Now, visualize yourself in pain because of your sadness and because of the shame and guilt you feel for harming others. Do not avoid feeling the intensity of your suffering, as you usually do. Consciously embrace the pain. With each in-breath, feel that suffering as if it were hot, thick, black smoke. Breathe it in deeply, but do not hold on to it. With each natural out-breath, imagine exhaling peace and tranquility, as if it were cool, fresh air.

4)   After several minutes of focusing on transforming your own suffering, visualize a person whom you harmed. Allow yourself to feel deeply the pain you caused them and your own remorse. Breathe in their suffering like black smoke, then, exhale a cooling peace. Sense your compassion as you breathe in their suffering, and your love as you breathe out peace and joy.

5)   Finally, imagine all the living creatures of the world and their suffering. Like you, all want to avoid sorrow and find happiness. Sense your oneness with the whole world. Inhale the suffering of the world and exhale happiness and peace.

You can use this exercise at any time, for even a few moments, with anyone you choose. It keeps you present to their suffering and helps develop empathy. The practice helps you nurture a compassionate, fearless heart, confident that the pain you encounter can never destroy you. In fact, the suffering, if embraced, can lead to new life.

In steps eight and nine you venture out of your self-contained depressed world. You recognize more clearly your freedom and choice. Either your mood or your values can guide your life. You consider carefully all your relationships and how you can improve them. Then you take action.

Dennis Ortman, Ph.D.

13

Out of the Shadows
Seeing Clearly

Step Ten: "Continued to take personal inventory and when we were wrong promptly admitted it."

"Repair the past, prepare the future.
Do not do today what you have always done."

—G.I. Gurdjieff

You walk deeper into the woods. You hoped you would eventually find your way out through this labyrinth, but your journey continues. Where and when will it end? As you proceed, the growing light does not make the way entirely clear. The shadows remain and mix with the light. It seems like twilight in that forest with twisted paths and trees. The colors stand out more. You can make out more shapes. The trees are not as alike as they seemed in the darkness. Everything begins to appear unique in its starkness.

Step ten invites you to make the inventory of the fourth step a regular practice. It continues the work of housecleaning in the present moment. *Emotions Anonymous* states: "In doing the fourth-step inventory we dealt honestly with our past so that we could free ourselves from it. This tenth-step inventory helps us deal with the present as we cope with daily living. Now that we are aware of our human imperfections, we realize we can easily fall back into our old ways of thinking and behaving" (p. 71-72).

You may have hoped that recovery would be a quick sprint to the finish line of relief from your depression. Unfortunately, it turned out to be a marathon, requiring more time, effort, and endurance than you expected. You may have had delightful moments in the zone, but often it was hard work. That should not be a surprise. You likely struggled with your depressive condition for many years and tried various strategies to find relief. Perhaps you hoped that working the steps would provide a quick and easy solution to your suffering. You hoped for a lasting cure. But none came.

Working the steps, you experienced the truth of AA's Serenity Prayer: "Lord, grant me the serenity to accept what I cannot change, the courage to change what I can, and the wisdom to know the difference." Paying close attention to your experience, you learned both your limits and your possibilities. You can only take responsibility for your own life, your own reactions, and your own behavior. In the process, you gain serenity, courage, and wisdom.

The Serenity Prayer resonates with a more ancient wisdom, that of the *Tao Te Ching*:

> **Knowing others is intelligence;**
> **knowing yourself is true wisdom.**
> **Mastering others is strength;**
> **mastering yourself is true power (33).**

These verses suggest the two-phase recovery that guides the AA program. The first is a step back to observe yourself closely, to learn wisdom. The second is a step forward in choosing to act, rather than react, gaining a sense of self-mastery. The Steps alternate between contemplation and action, a graceful back and forth movement. The goal is progress, not perfection.

AVOIDING THE SELF-APPRAISAL

Your depression may interfere with your making a realistic, regular self-appraisal. You may judge yourself harshly, become impatient, or tend to give up the effort.

Mallory, judging himself harshly:

"I hear my father's voice in my head constantly, 'Don't do this. Don't do that. You shouldn't do this. You should do that.' It just about drives me crazy. I call it 'the Judge.' I know the judge's expectations are unrealistic and harsh, but I can't ignore them. I'm always monitoring myself and never feeling like I'm measuring up. What's worse is that I can't just judge myself. I'm monitoring everyone in my life. They sense my disappointment and resent it. I can understand that and feel guilty about it."

Depression has been described as anger turned inward. Its face is that of a harsh judge. You judge yourself mercilessly and become a prosecutor. Unfortunately, the anger and judgment do not stay inward. You hold others up to your unrealistic standards and prosecute them too. When they criticize you, you become a defense attorney, even though secretly you agree with them. The severity of your standards prevents you from being a fair, impartial judge of yourself.

Lizzie, impatient for a cure:

"How much more can I take? I've suffered depression my whole life and been in treatment. I've tried more medications than I can count. One works for a while and I feel hopeful. Then suddenly, it stops working. The doctor prescribes another that,

again, helps for a while. We start the routine over. I've been involved in counseling, both individual and group. I've read every self-help book available. The doctors tell me I have a relapsing illness. Sometimes it's just so discouraging."

Patience can be in short supply when you struggle with a chronic illness such as depression. The pain can be nearly intolerable at times. You may want to give up. Hopelessness is a close companion. The approach of the Twelve Steps that invites you to embrace your illness and learn from it can seem so unrealistic and cruel. You do not believe that you can learn patience, compassion, and wisdom when you are so desperate for a cure.

Cynthia, wanting to forget:

"I've suffered so many losses in life, I just want to forget. When my boyfriend died in an auto accident, I wanted to give up on life. I had many suicidal thoughts. I just wanted to die to escape the pain. I've been to therapy and taken medications, but they never really helped. Only one thing has helped. I smoke marijuana every day. It helps me forget and get by."

Your depression makes you want to withdraw into passivity. After fighting your painful emotions, you may feel defeated and want to give up. "What's the use?" you tell yourself. The path of working with your thoughts and feelings requires effort, constant vigilance, and disciplined action. When you have a lifelong struggle with your moods, you may become lazy and refuse to make the effort. As AA constantly reminds its members, "You have to work the program." There are no quick fixes. There are no short cuts. However, you will undoubtedly have bright moments and feel a sense of accomplishment.

EXAMINATION OF CONSCIOUSNESS

Step ten begins by recommending a regular practice of the fourth step. But instead of taking a "moral inventory," it suggests a "personal inventory." Limiting yourself to a moral inventory may indulge your inner critic, which engages in routine fault-finding missions. Your self-esteem suffers. In contrast, the personal inventory is a deeper examination of consciousness that recognizes both strengths and weaknesses. It balances your tendency toward negative self-judgment. It also goes deeper than the surface of your thoughts, feelings, and behaviors, inviting you to glimpse answers to these questions: Who are you? Where are you going? What would fulfill you?

WHAT: EXAMINE YOUR REACTION CHAIN

What do you pay attention to in your personal inventory? Your addiction to depression does not possess you all at once, full blown. You may have been born with a biological predisposition to a mood disorder. With the accumulated experience of losses, your depression deepens. It may come and go. You may have periods of calm and sudden relapses that seem to come out of the blue. The moods overtake you like a storm. But if you pay close attention, you will notice the rising dark clouds in the blue sky of your life. The clouds increase and darken the sky, become more threatening, and eventually erupt in a terrible storm.

You can work with your moods by observing closely the signs and symptoms of the rising storm. If you can interrupt the chain reaction of growing distress, you can protect yourself from drowning in the storm. A saying from an unknown source (1) describes the links in the reaction chain within your mind and their connections. I have added two links:

> Watch your physical sensations; they become emotions.
> Watch your emotions; they become thoughts.
> Watch your thoughts; they become words.
> Watch your words; they become actions.
> Watch your actions; they become habits.
> Watch your habits; they become character.
> Watch your character; it becomes your destiny.

When your mood is changing, take a zoom lens look at your experience. Notice the unique way that you experience depression so you can recognize the emerging pattern of reacting more quickly the next time it occurs:

Body Sensations: Your body holds the pain of the losses you experience and never forgets. Your muscles constrict, preparing for fighting, fleeing, or freezing. Where do you feel tension most? Do you become agitated or numbed? Do you feel drained of energy?

Emotions: The four main emotional groups are sad, mad, glad, and scared. What combination do you feel mostly? Notice their fluctuations, their ebb and flow, and variations in intensity. You may detect subtle feelings within feelings, such as shame, guilt, envy, pride, resentment, greed, lust, and so forth. You may miss feelings of delight, elation, gaiety, enjoyment, pleasure, and so forth. What is your predominant feeling? How much do you crave approval, love, accomplishments, perfection, and so forth? What losses disturb you most?

Thoughts: Based on past experiences, you spontaneously interpret events as favorable, unfavorable, or neutral. These interpretations interact with your spontaneous emotional reactions. When you are depressed, the thoughts run in a negative direction with unrealistic expectations. What automatic negative thoughts arise in your current situation? Notice the worries, regrets, blaming, criticism, and so forth. What expectations do you entertain for yourself and others? How realistic are they? What happy memories and blessings of loved ones do you overlook?

Words: Your thoughts take shape in words both inside and outside yourself. What internal dialogue is going on in your head? How do you speak to other people? What beliefs about yourself, relationships, and the world do you express?

Actions: Actions arise from impulses deep within you. They are also shaped by your feelings, motives, and thoughts. How do you treat yourself and others? If you are depressed, you tend to neglect your basic needs. As AA observes with the acronym HALT: "Don't be hungry, angry, lonely, or tired." Do you care for yourself properly?

Habits: Repeated actions become habits. What habitual patterns of feeling, thinking, and behaving do you observe? If you are depressed, you tend to avoid painful feelings by distracting or numbing yourself. Do you engage in any addictive behaviors to self-medicate your pain?

Character: You naturally reflect on your life experience and tell yourself stories about yourself. The stories make sense of the chaos of your experience and give you an identity. What stories do you tell yourself about who you are? Those who are depressed tend to identify with their depressed role in life. They may see themselves as victims, losers, or helpless children. How do you see yourself?

Destiny: Your choices have consequences, some foreseen and others not, creating your character and destiny. The values you choose give direction to your life and shape your destiny. What do you value? What are your priorities in life? What is the gap between the way you would like your life to be and the way it is? You can change your destiny by aligning your life more with your values than the dictates of your mood.

WHO: THE OBSERVING SELF

Who examines your life in making your personal inventory? The answer may seem obvious. "I do," you tell yourself. But who is the "I" that is doing the observing. You cannot perceive that "I" directly. That would be making it an object of your viewing, like an eyeball looking at itself. There is no place to stand from which to observe that "I" objectively. There is, then, some "I" behind the act of observing and reflecting that you cannot observe. It transcends your looking.

We can call this subjective, transcending "I" your observing self. You sense its invisible presence in the act of watching the chain of reaction. These sensations, feelings, and thoughts come from you, yet are not you as a person. Science, psychology, and ancient wisdom testify to this observing self.

Science tells us that inner space mirrors outer space. Outer space is open and nearly without limits. It contains countless planets, stars, and galaxies that are in constant motion and separated by light years of space. According to the "Big Bang" theory, the universe is expanding to unknown limits. In a similar way, viewing matter through a microscope, we see atoms composed of nuclei surrounded by whirling electrons, which are like planets orbiting the sun. The atoms bind together to form molecules. The molecules join together to form objects, like galaxies of matter. What appears to be solid mass is really composed of moving objects in an empty space. The bodies are held within an expanding emptiness.

Psychology tells us that the human mind mirrors the material universe. Thoughts, feelings, and sensations are like planets and stars moving through empty space, which is the consciousness. They are in constant motion, always changing, never the same. These mental objects join together to form fixed ideas and beliefs, like galaxies of ideas. Consciousness holds all these mental objects without being defined by them. They are merely self-created objects floating in your mental space. Furthermore, consciousness, like space, is expanding to unknown limits. Your observing self is really consciousness open to all reality and not limited by its contents.

Ancient wisdom tells us about the openness of mind. The *Tao Te Ching*, composed 25 centuries ago, teaches the usefulness of the empty mind using comparisons:

We join spokes together in a wheel,
but it is the center hole
that makes the wagon move.

**We shape clay into a pot,
but it is the emptiness inside
that holds whatever we want.**

**We hammer wood for a house,
but it is the inner space
that makes it livable.**

**We work with being,
but non-being is what we use (11).**

The vastness and openness of consciousness is like the center hole of a wheel, the emptiness inside a pot, and the inner space of a house. It makes life workable and livable, if we only recognize and use its power. Using your awareness, you sense your basic goodness, innate sanity, and natural bravery.

Another image. The stream of consciousness flows like a river. Objects emerge from its depths. These are our sensations, feelings, and thoughts. These objects come from the river, but they are not the river itself. The river's waters come from and return to the ocean, its vast source. The ocean is God, Ultimate Reality, the Source. Our consciousness participates in the Divine and can be called Spirit.

Why is it important to be aware of the observing self? The awareness releases the energy of the Higher Power within. It frees you from the bondage of the fixed ideas and automatic reactions that enslave you. You are able to fully engage in the immediate experience of the moment, rather than living in the artificial world of your ideas. What is the benefit?

- Your emotional reactions of sadness, fear, anger, and disappointment do not touch your core. You can get off the emotional roller coaster.

- You see the emptiness of your nagging self-criticism, inflated expectations, and distorted negative beliefs. You can withdraw your faith from these misguided ideas.

- You recognize the stories you tell yourself as creative fiction. You can rewrite your stories to reflect your current experience of yourself.

- Your engrained habits of feeling, thinking, and behaving lose their hold on you. You feel free to give them up and transform them.

HOW AND WHEN: THE SPOT-CHECK INVENTORY

In the midst of an emotional disturbance, the Steps/Traditions book recommends a spot-check inventory. As much as you hate it, feeling emotionally distressed can be a privileged moment to learn about yourself. You experience, in the moment, your vulnerability and your programmed reactions of coping. The spot check is an invitation to get out of your head and engage in a present moment experience. You turn the spotlight on yourself. It requires the exercise of many skills, which become stronger in their use: "In all these situations we need self-restraint, honest analysis of what is involved, a willingness to forgive when the fault is ours, and an equal willingness to forgive when the fault is elsewhere" (p. 91). The more you sincerely practice this inward look, the more proficient you become.

How do you make this inventory? An ancient Eastern text, *The Way of the Bodhisattva* (2), proposes a method. It suggests a practice to stop, look, and listen to yourself before acting. The practice is called, "Remaining like a log." Self-control begins by learning to take a pause between an arising urge and the automatic behavior. Shantideva, the author, advises:

> **When the urge arises in the mind**
> **to feelings of desire or wrathful hate,**
> **do not act! Be silent, do not speak!**
> **And like a log of wood be sure to stay.**

When an urge arises, such as sadness, fear, anger, or any other emotional reaction, there are four moments when you can intervene and gain control of yourself:

Before a thought is formed in the mind, the reaction begins with an initial perception. Some sight, sound, physical sensation, or memory causes discomfort. Awareness of this initial discomfort can prevent an emotional avalanche from gaining momentum.

Next, be aware of the spontaneous thoughts that accompany the discomfort. You may be unaware of these emerging thoughts, which express some negative interpretation of the perception. Simply observing these thoughts keeps them from gaining power over your mind.

If you ignore the subtle thoughts that accompany your emotional reaction, your emotions will intensify and be prolonged. It is still not too late to catch these arising thoughts with your mind's eye and stop the avalanche of emotion. You can observe the pattern of these gathering thoughts and recognize the negative bias they express.

Finally, there is a moment when the urge leads to action. You can train yourself to stop and think before taking action. You can interrupt the automatic chain reaction that has formed into an addictive habit. You can stop to consider what you value and how you want to act, making a free choice. Even in the face of an intense emotion that seems overwhelming, you are not as helpless as you think.

Penelope, sensitive to anger:

"When my husband raises his voice I become very upset. I tell him he's yelling at me. He insists that he's not angry or yelling. My stomach is in knots and I feel a sense of panic when it happens. Then I stop and think before I react. I know where my sensitivity to yelling comes from. My father had a terrible temper and yelled at us kids. Sometimes he became violent. I was terrified and just wanted to run and hide. I feel the same way as an adult when I sense any anger in anyone."

BREAKING BAD, MAKING GOOD

The purpose of the personal inventory is to prepare you for action. You make a firm purpose of amendment. Then you take Steps to transform your bad habits into good ones. Recognizing your automatic reactions, you consciously choose to let your values guide your life.

Change requires the three As: awareness, acceptance, and action. In making your personal inventory, you become more aware of your chain of reactions to various situations. You gain some understanding of your automatic tendencies, your weaknesses, and your strengths. You realize that what you consider unbreakable habits are not as solid as you think. Furthermore, what you value becomes clearer as you notice your reactions to various losses. You have a choice between your automatic reactions and your values.

Accepting, rather than rejecting, yourself releases the energy for you to effect change in a valued direction. It is the energy of compassion, which comes from the heart. Your self-defeating habits of feeling, thinking, and acting cause you and others suffering. You behave like a wounded child who has suffered many losses in life. Your inner child is crying out to be embraced with love, not scolded for its shortcomings. Acknowledge, with tenderness, that your faults were misguided ways of compensating for a void you felt in your life. You can fill that emptiness with love, which will express itself in valued living.

Now you can take action. What do you want to do? Where do you want to go with your life? Your depression makes you resistant to change. Change only means painful losses, endings, and dying. It takes a courageous leap of faith into the unknown to imagine gains, beginnings, and new life. There is no shortcut or easy way. Breaking bad habits and creating new ones will require you to do something different. That means pushing yourself beyond your comfort zone and tolerating the discomfort. Remember that the anxiety you feel in doing something new may be distressful, but it will not harm you. Staying stuck in your depressed mood will.

I often ask my depressed patients, "What would you do if you were not depressed?" Most have some idea of how catering to their mood holds them back. I then ask, "Why would you give your mood so much power over your life?" Make the commitment to let what you value, rather than your moods, be your guide. Think about what you can do differently so you are not controlled by your depressed habits. For example:

- If your depression makes you withdraw from socializing and other activities, challenge your passive tendencies. In the process, you will become a more confident and generous person.

- If you become preoccupied with your physical and emotional pain, learn to forget yourself for a moment and reach out to others who are suffering. You will gain compassion.

- If you freeze into anxious indecision, accept the lack of guarantees for being right and the tentativeness of every decision. Making decisions in the face of fear and doubt will increase your courage.

- If you are a perfectionist, let go of your unrealistic expectations, live in the present moment, and find moderation and peace.

- If automatic pessimistic thoughts and judgments occupy your mind, learn to confront them with your rational, wise mind. Your reward will be wisdom.

- If you attack yourself mercilessly for being inadequate and worthless, learn to relax your inner critic. You will learn humility, kindness, and gentleness in the process.

- If thoughts of helplessness and hopelessness dominate your thinking, see their emptiness and push on regardless. Strength and determination will be the fruit of your labors.

- If your temper has the best of you, learn to take a time out and see things from a different perspective. You have the opportunity to develop patience.

- If worries about coming catastrophes monopolize your thinking, see their emptiness and resolve to let them go. Serenity and tranquility will be the consequence.

- If you despair about the future and give up trying, stop to consider the consequences and redouble your efforts. Then you will discover an unsuspected zeal, strength, and hope within you.

- If you feel sorry for yourself, look around and notice others who are suffering. Your heart will become compassionate.

By being aware of your depressive tendencies and consciously acting against them, you replace unwholesome habits of living with healthy ones.

Sidney, working with his moods:

"I've been depressed my whole life and learned through trial and error what I have to do to take care of myself. I know I need to keep taking my medication. When I stopped, it was a disaster. I hate the winters. I always feel worse that time of year. I can't escape the darkness. When the mood hits, all I want to do is sleep. I know that's not good for me. So I push myself. What helps most is to go with the church group to the nursing home and talk with the residents. That always lifts my mood."

Lance, preventing relapse:

"I grew up in an alcoholic family. I understand why I became depressed, because I felt so neglected as a child. I drank heavily for a while, but now have been sober ten years. My family is still drinking. I don't see them often, but during the holidays I want to keep some connection. Before going to a family party, I prepare myself so I don't become depressed or drink. My wife is at my side. We talk about having an escape plan. When I feel too overwhelmed by the chaos, we agreed that we would make an excuse and leave. My sanity depends on having relapse prevention plans."

PARADOX OF DYING AND LIVING

Hooked on depression, you are familiar with dying. You already feel dead inside. You lack vitality, clinging to painful losses. Because of the intensity of the pain, you may even long for death or consider suicide. "I'm already dead. What difference would it make if I take my life?" you may tell yourself.

Step ten challenges you with another paradox: "From dying comes new life." Instead of hating your life as it is, it invites you to embrace it with love, even with all the pain. Your pain can be the way to new life. Jesus said, "I solemnly assure you, unless the grain of wheat falls to the earth and dies, it remains just a grain of wheat. But if it dies, it produces much fruit" (John 12:24). How can the painful dying of depression lead to new life?

Depression can be a gift if it leads you to look more deeply into your life and ask, "What needs to die in me? What needs to come to life?" Your depressed mind focuses on the ending, the loss, the dying, but does not consider the new beginning and life.

In your recovery, the unhealthy habits of the old self die through a gradual process of recognizing them and letting them go. Attachments keep you stuck and need to be dropped like the dead weight they are. The energy of your vices does not simply evaporate. Instead, it is transformed, through effort and grace, into life-giving habits. Your willfulness, being preoccupied with yourself, becomes a willingness to embrace others in love.

Just as you cannot force the grain of wheat to grow, you cannot create a new life for yourself through sheer will power. You can cultivate the soil through disciplined practice. However, the fruits of a liberated life flourish through surrendering to a Higher Power that dwells both within and beyond you. Will power, the desire to have absolute control over your life, must die for you to be free and genuinely happy.

PRACTICE: AN EVENING INVENTORY

The Steps/Traditions book recommends, in addition to the spot-check inventory, a regular evening inventory. It suggests drawing up "a balance sheet for the day," not only what is done in red ink, but also in black ink. Your anxiety draws you to the negative. An accurate balance sheet of your life must include the positive, what you have done right, for a more balanced perspective.

A Japanese practice called "Naikan," which means "looking inside," can be helpful for this balanced accounting at the end of the day (3). The practice invites you to reflect on the past twenty-four hours of your day and ask yourself three questions: 1) What have I received? 2) What have I given? 3) What difficulties have I caused?

What have I received?

Your depressive instinct focuses on what is missing, not on what is present. Your glass is always half empty, never half full. You see the void, not the abundance. Because you pay so much attention to what you do not have, or fear losing, you ignore what you already have. Your life is full, and you do not even recognize it. At the end of the day, pause to reflect on all the good things you received. Contemplate the simple pleasures: kindnesses from those you encountered, a joyful moment with the family, a call from a friend.

Noticing your blessings can inspire an attitude of gratitude to offset your preoccupation with things going wrong.

What have I given?

When you are depressed, you withdraw to nurse your wounds. You may expect others to adjust their lives to your sensitivities. Self-preoccupation and a sense of entitlement may creep into your life. To confront this tendency, it is important to consider what you did for others. Note even the simple things: a friendly greeting at the store, listening to a friend's troubles, doing your work with a joyful heart.

Noticing your own spontaneous generosity can increase your self-confidence that you have much to offer.

What difficulties have I caused?

Your harsh self-critic can make you either exaggerate your faults or hide them in shame. True humility invites you to see yourself accurately and recognize the impact of your behavior on others. At the end of the day, honestly admit to yourself how you may have harmed others by what you have done or not done for them. Perhaps you overlooked opportunities to show love. Allow feelings of remorse to rise in your heart. That will motivate you to find a way to repair the damage, both to yourself and the other person.

The ongoing effort to transform your unhealthy habits to beneficial ones releases a new energy. You feel free and alive. Your heart is open to embrace the world. Seeds of joy begin to blossom.

Grateful Abundance
Living Fully Now

*Step Eleven: "Sought through prayer and meditation
to improve our conscious contact with God, as we understood Him,
praying only for knowledge of His will for us and the power to carry it out."*

"If the only prayer you say your entire life is 'Thank you,' that would suffice."

—Meister Eckhart

Your longing for the light increases as you proceed on your journey. The darkness is not total. You see flashes of light regularly and rare spotlight moments when the whole forest appears bathed in light. Your confidence grows. Despite your fears, you know the light overshadows the darkness. You see your way more clearly, including all the obstacles. The woods come alive with color, and you tell yourself, "What a wonderful world!"

Step eleven expresses the second major theme of the Steps: "trust God." It invites you to continue deepening your relationship with your Higher Power, with God, that you began in the second and third Steps. A thread of prayer also runs through all the Steps, the spirit of the Serenity Prayer.

The Steps/Traditions book underlines the benefits, and necessity, of prayer for your continued growth: "We want the good that is in us all, even in the worst of us, to flower and grow. Most certainly we shall need bracing air and an abundance of food. But first of all we shall want sunlight; nothing much can grow in the dark. Meditation is our step out into the sun" (p. 98). Actually, it is a step into the present moment with full awareness.

Because of your difficulty adjusting to change and the accompanying losses, you look for some anchor, "a still point in the turning world." The AA program suggests three: God, the present moment, and the group. But you may find yourself clinging to your mood instead.

OBSESSING AND HOPELESS

Depression stops you dead in your tracks. To cope with the pain of sorrow, you withdraw within yourself to nurse the wound. Life is too much for you. You need to get off the merry-go-round for a moment to make some mental and emotional adjustments. Your grieving can open your heart to absorbing and accepting the loss. The acceptance, then, frees you for new life.

Your depression makes you a natural contemplative. You want to be alone, quiet, and still. You withdraw from the maddening crowd and all the hustle and bustle. Prayer and meditation on the meaning of your life can spontaneously happen. However, when you become stuck in your mood, you may be unable to concentrate enough to pray. Your obsessing and sense of hopelessness may interfere.

Reggie, lost in his thoughts:

"When I'm depressed, I just want to be left alone. I want to sleep, but my mind keeps me awake. I can't relax, hard as I try. My mind jumps around. I think about the past, all the things that went wrong, and all my regrets. I think about how miserable I am. Then, my mind jumps to the future. I worry about what is going to happen to me and my family. Back and forth my mind goes. I try to pray, but it's useless. I can't even concentrate enough to say the rosary and really mean it."

Absorbed in your pain, you cannot think about anything else. You brood about what has gone wrong and will go wrong in your life. Negative thoughts imprison you in a mental cave, and there is no escape. Your mind runs around in circles, bumping into the walls. There is no sunlight, only darkness. There is no stillness, only noise. The mental confusion interferes with you quieting your mind and body enough for prayer or meditation.

Hilary, living without hope:

"Whatever can go wrong in life has happened to me. My parents died when I was young. My husband left me for another woman. And I recently lost my job. I don't see any reason to go on. I think often about suicide, but I don't have the courage to do it. I feel so hopeless. My friends encourage me to pray and assure me God will help me. A good God wouldn't allow me to suffer this much. Where was God when I needed Him?"

Hopelessness and despair often accompany depression. Doom and gloom dominate your life. The future seems empty. Your world is bleak. Your pessimistic attitude closes your mind and heart to the possibility of any goodness that God could offer. It interferes with the receptive openness needed for prayer.

HOW TO PRAY

Prayer and meditation are difficult for anyone living in our restless culture that spawns so many addictions. The various religious/spiritual groups in our culture, including AA, take up the challenge of calling us to pray. We learn to pray in different ways, according to our religious background, temperament, and season of life.

I was raised Roman Catholic. Observing my own spiritual history, I noticed different ways of praying at various times in my life.

SAYING PRAYERS

My parents first taught me to pray as a young child. Each night before going to bed, my mom or dad would kneel down with me at the bedside. They taught me to make the sign of the cross and fold my hands. Then together we said: "Angel of God, my guardian dear, to whom God's love commits me here. Ever this night be at my side, to light and guard, to rule and guide." Next, we asked for God's blessings on various people and ended with the sign of the cross. That bedside prayer inspired confidence in me that God loved me, watched over me, and protected me from any dangers.

In grade school, the nuns taught me more prayers to recite. We learned the "Our Father," "Hail Mary," and "Glory Be," prayers taken from the Scriptures. We recited them carefully in class and put them together to pray the rosary. Reciting these prayers, I gained a sense of belonging to a faith community with a solid tradition. Initially, I merely memorized the words, but gradually, I let their meaning penetrate my heart. I felt closeness with God.

TALKING WITH GOD

Attending high school retreats, I was taught another way of praying. Instead of using the community's words, I was encouraged to speak to God from my heart in my own words. "Be spontaneous. Tell God whatever you are feeling. Speak to Him from your heart, as you would a close friend," my religion teachers urged me. I experienced God as an intimate Friend and sought a personal relationship with Him. In prayer, I expressed to God my deepest desires and secrets that I would tell no one else. He was my Confidant.

LISTENING FROM THE HEART

While in the college seminary, we each had a spiritual director and regular conferences. The spiritual director instructed us about different forms of praying. What impressed me most at this time was a shift in my prayer from speaking to listening. Hearing what God was saying to me in the depths of my heart was more important than what I was telling Him. I learned the importance of being still and silent. I also learned to read the words of Scripture slowly and reflectively, letting the words penetrate to my core. "Be still and know that I am God" (Psalm 46:10) became the theme of my daily meditation. I came to appreciate God's mysterious, unshakable presence in my life.

BEING STILL

Solitude, silence, and stillness have become the hallmarks of my prayer and meditation for the last several years. Jesus' response to his disciples' inquiring about how to pray makes more sense to me now. He taught, "When you pray, go to your inner room, close the door and pray to your Father in secret. And your Father, who sees in secret, will reward you" (Matt. 6:6). The inner room is within me, where God is closer to me than I am to myself. I sense Him living and praying through me. I try to live the words of St. Paul, urging his congregation to "pray constantly." My prayer and life are not so separate. Frequently, I pause during the day to be consciously aware of God's enduring Presence.

I looked outside my Christian upbringing to the Eastern traditions that promoted the value of contemplation centuries before Christianity. Their wisdom showed a path to serenity and peace similar to the way of Christ. For example, the *Tao Te Ching* advocates emptying the mind to find peace:

> **Empty your mind of all thoughts.**
> **Let your heart be at peace.**
> **Watch the turmoil of beings,**
> **but contemplate their return.**
> **Each separate being in the universe**
> **returns to the common source.**
> **Returning to the source is serenity.**
> **If you don't realize the source,**
> **you stumble in confusion and sorrow (22).**

ANCHORING IN THE PRESENT MOMENT

Whatever way you choose to pray, it anchors you in the present moment. Your depression flings you to the past with all its regrets and to the future with all its worries. You become lost in your time travel thoughts. Instead, prayer brings you back to the experience of the Divine in the present moment. It is here, in this place, in this time, in these circumstances, that you encounter God, your Higher Power, and nowhere else. The present is the point of intersection between time and eternity. Living the moment, you contemplate the common Source from which all life flows and returns.

Thich Nhat Hanh, the renowned Buddhist monk, founded a movement called "Engaged Buddhism." He grew up in Vietnam and protested the war, calling both sides to reconciliation. He was nominated for the Nobel Peace Prize for his efforts. Hanh believed that true meditation enabled a person to become more fully engaged in life, which included the political and social arena. He affirmed that our true home is in the here and now. This is the place of our happiness and peace. He taught a simple meditation practice centered on the breath (1):

> **"Breathing in, I calm my body.**
> **Breathing out, I smile.**
> **Dwelling in the present moment**
> **I know this is a wonderful moment."**

ENLARGING YOUR CONSCIOUSNESS

Your depressed mind gravitates to what is missing in your life, to absence, to past losses. It is fueled by pain, anger, and disappointment. The prayerful mind, in contrast, focuses on what is present, on abundance. You anchor your consciousness to the present moment. It experiences wholeness and draws from its Source, the God of goodness and mercy. You have a choice of which mind to cultivate, either the depressed mind of disappointment or the prayerful mind of satisfaction.

The depressed mind has its own operating system:

- It focuses on how your life fails to meet your expectations.

- It focuses on what is missing, the gap between what you want and what you get.

- It engages in scarcity thinking, on not having enough or being good enough.

- It results in suffering, depression, and disappointment.

Or you can follow the prayerful mind with its expanded consciousness:

- It focuses on what life is offering, on the gifts being received.

- It embraces the fullness of experience, excluding nothing.

- It engages in abundance thinking, on the goodness already possessed.

- It results in happiness, gratitude, and generosity.

MAKING GOD YOUR ANCHOR

When depressed, the greatest loss you suffer is the loss of your true self. Many of my depressed patients lament, "I don't know myself. I don't know what I want in life." Through all the tumultuous changes in their lives, they have lost the inner compass of their identity. They feel disconnected from themselves, others, and God. They feel adrift in life without an anchor.

Working step ten, you became more aware of your observing self, which is open, spacious consciousness. Science, psychology, and ancient wisdom offered insights for understanding the self. Religion also can provide a vehicle to know yourself. It alerts us to the intimate connection between God and us. Thomas Merton, the well-known monk of Gethsemane Abbey, eloquently stated: "Therefore there is only one problem on which all my existence, my peace and my happiness depend: to discover myself in discovering God. If I find Him, I will find myself, and if I find my true self, I will find Him" (2).

Religion tells us that God dwells at the deepest core of our observing self. Consciousness can be named Spirit. We are made in the image and likeness of God, sharing His life. Of course, you can understand this divine-human connection in many ways, according to your own preferred understanding. God may be for you a Someone, a Personal Presence with different names. Or it may be a Something larger than yourself: Creative Intelligence,

Reality, Life Force, Universal Spirit, the Source, and so forth. The word religion means "to bind again." It affirms that we participate in a Reality larger than our small selves that connects us with the whole universe and others.

There is both a danger and an opportunity in seeing ourselves as divine. Bill Wilson, the cofounder of AA, clearly stated in the "Big Book" the danger for anyone addiction-prone: "Selfishness—self-centeredness! That, we think, is the root of our troubles...First of all, we had to quit playing God. It didn't work" (p. 62). Our ego-driven life wants to make us the center of the universe and have the world revolve around us. We want to be special, worshipped, all-knowing and all-powerful.

However, there is another deeper desire that comes from our true self, to be more god-like. As St. Paul writes, "Be imitators of God as his dear children. Follow the way of love, even as Christ loved you" (Ephesians 5:1-2). The higher calling of the true self is to live a life of virtue, of selfless love. It is an invitation to choose a value-directed life, rather than be driven by sadness and fear.

This larger consciousness, anchored in a confidence of Divine Presence, has a direct impact on how you live and relate to others. There's a Buddhist parable that shows this truth:

One day, as the Buddha was sitting under a tree, a young, trim soldier walked by. He looked at the Buddha, noted his full girth, and said, "You look like a pig!" The Buddha looked up calmly and responded, "You look like God!" Startled by the comment, the soldier asked, "Why do you say that I look like God?" The Buddha replied, "We don't really see what's outside ourselves. We see what's inside us and project it out. I sit under this tree all day and contemplate God. So when I look out, that's what I see. And you must be thinking about other things."

We see others as we see ourselves. When you are trapped in depression, what do you see? If you view yourself a victim, you will see others as persecutors and resent them. Your anger will make you their persecutors. If you view yourself a loser, you encourage others to treat you that way. You invite others to treat you the way you treat yourself. If you imagine yourself a helpless child, you will expect and demand others to care for you. You will become dependent on them and resent your lack of independence. If you acknowledge your God-given greatness, you will act with a magnanimous heart.

DISCERNING GOD'S WILL (YOUR TRUE DESIRES)

When you pray in solitude and silence, you discover the answers to two questions: Who am I? What should I do? You acquire knowledge of your true self, hidden beneath your moods. You also become empowered to live according to the deepest desires of your real self.

Ancient Christian wisdom proclaims, "The glory of God is the person full alive." There is a direct correspondence between what God wants and what satisfies our deepest desires. The difficulty is that in any given situation we are not sure what we really want. Competing desires vie for attention. How do you decide? What do you really want? What is in your best interests to do?

Lorraine, feeling lonely:

"My husband died a year ago suddenly of a heart attack. We were married 40 years and did everything together. Now I feel so lonely. I can't stand being alone. We used to go to Florida for the winter, but I can't go there now. It only brings back memories of him and how much I miss him. I used to enjoy socializing and playing the piano. I don't do anything now. My family tries to get me to go out. I just sit home and brood. I don't know what to do. I don't know what will make me happy."

Depression creates a crisis for you. It is both a danger and an opportunity. You can stay stuck, wallowing in self-pity. Or you can explore its meaning, learn its wisdom, and create a new life for yourself. Your mood invites you to make a decision for either death or life. Essentially, you are seeking to discern God's will for you in this life situation. How do you decide? Three issues arise in the discernment process:

WHAT IS THE QUESTION?

Working the Steps, you discovered that your mood is not your problem as you assumed. It is only a symptom of a deeper problem. To discover the root problem you need to embrace your mood and enter into the heart of its darkness. Your depression is telling you that something is not working in your life. Somehow you have gone off track. Your painful mood is really your true self crying out to be heard. Remember that the word depressed means that some life force within you is being pressed down and needs to surface. You feel so dead because your natural vitality is being suppressed.

The depression gives you a clue to what is missing in your life. Sadness is a natural reaction to loss. Your mood poses several questions for you to consider:

- What do you miss so desperately in your life in this moment?

- What life task might you be avoiding by your depression?

- Where do you need to grow up?

- How are you neglecting to take care of yourself?

WHAT IS INVOLVED?

The emotional pain creates a sense of urgency to explore its meaning. An effective way to discover the meaning of your mood is to make a careful personal inventory. Follow closely your chains of reaction to uncover your habitual patterns of feeling, thinking, and behaving. Notice what losses you are most sensitive to. That sensitivity reveals your attachments, what you cling to with the false belief that their attainment will make you happy. You will observe the mask you wear to support the pursuit of these desires. You may notice an exhausting chase after money, love, status, power, approval, success, achievements, perfection, and so forth. Consider the gains and losses in their pursuit.

Your personal inventory will also lead you to explore the deeper longings disguised in these distorted desires. Your true self yearns to be heard and express itself. It expresses itself in your values, the pursuits that make your life full and meaningful.

- What character defects, distorted desires, do you need to let go?

- What do you value most in life?

- What makes you feel alive?

WHAT IS YOUR RESPONSE?

Despite your feelings of helplessness, you are born free. You have a choice. You can choose to let your life be directed by your mood and the mind of disappointment. Or you can lead a value-directed life, letting your mind of abundance guide you.

In this concrete situation, consider what your depression is asking of you and what changes you need to make. Reflect on the proposed action in the context of your life. Step back and look at the flow of your life up to this point. Ask yourself if this decision is more consistent or inconsistent with your life history. Consider what values have guided your life and whether the proposed action is compatible with those values. For example, you may recognize a lack of balance in your life and the need to recommit yourself to your partner, to work, or to your health. Allow something new to emerge in your life and observe its trajectory.

After this thorough review, consulting with your wise mind, make a tentative decision. Observe how sitting with the decision feels. Notice especially the flow of energy, whether it feels more or less blocked. Persistent turmoil, agitation, and lethargy indicate that you are not yet ready to make the decision. A sustained feeling of inner peace and energy normally follows a wise decision, even though you may feel some anxiety in carrying it out. Feelings of peace, courage, strength, and consolation emerge from following the guidance of your true self. Feelings of anxiety, sadness, confusion, and inner disturbance arise from letting your false self-control your decision-making.

- Does your decision bring peace and renewed energy?

- Are you made larger or smaller by the decision?

- Are you living your own life or that of another?

FINDING AN ANCHOR IN THE GROUP

Bill Wilson acknowledged two ways of accessing your Higher Power: through prayer and through the fellowship of AA. He stated: "But there exists among us a fellowship, a friendliness, and an understanding which is indescribably wonderful. We are like passengers of a great liner the moment after the rescue from shipwreck when camaraderie, joyousness and democracy pervade the vessel from steerage to Captain's table" (3).

Your depression makes you want to isolate yourself. The last thing you want to do is join a group and interact with others. It takes so much energy. Plus, you feel so bad about yourself. Perhaps pushing yourself to associate with others will energize you and release a Power buried under the ruble of your illness.

Our culture promotes a rugged individualism that may be detrimental to our wellbeing. Even in matters of the Spirit, Americans want to go on their own. Since the time of Bill Wilson, Americans have described themselves more as "spiritual," privately searching, than "religious," belonging to a church. Even though consistently over the years ninety-two percent claim they believe in God, only twenty percent of adults and thirty percent of those under thirty years of age are affiliated with a church. Only twenty percent attend services weekly, even though three quarters pray regularly (4).

The founders of the great religions were all spiritual searchers. Yet they all decided to gather a community around them. After encountering Yahweh in the burning bush, Moses gathered the Jewish people and led them out of slavery from Egypt. The Buddha became enlightened under the bodhi tree and rejoined his five companions, sharing with them the four noble truths. After his baptism in the Jordan, Jesus called twelve apostles and began preaching the good news. Muhammad received God's revelation alone in a cave, shared the message with his family, and called forth a community to surrender to Allah.

Organized religious communities of all denominations have survived for centuries. Meanwhile, governments have come and gone and civilizations have arisen and fallen with regularity. It seems miraculous that churches have survived the corruption of their leadership, countless scandals, and the hypocrisy of so many members. Even all the religious wars have not destroyed them. What is the secret? Perhaps Gamaliel's advice to his Jewish cohorts regarding the followers of Jesus rings true: "Let them alone. If their purpose or activity is human in its origin, it will destroy itself. If, on the other hand, it comes from God, you will not be able to destroy them without fighting God himself" (Acts 5: 38-39).

Why is joining a support group and/or religious community so important for you if you are depressed? Your spiritual journey of recovery is a perilous one. The urge to isolate and become self-absorbed with your pain is strong. Being with others, especially those on a similar journey, can help heal you. Freud observed that love heals. You cannot love alone. You need others to love and be loved. Gathering together can release the power of love and create a place for the mutual expression of healing love. In the Christian tradition, God is love, a community of Persons united in perfect love, called the Trinity.

Samantha, seeking a place to belong:

"I've never felt like I belonged. That has made me feel lonely and depressed. When I'm depressed, I stay home, feel lonelier and become more depressed. In therapy, I realized this vicious cycle and its effects on my mood. So I decided to join a Yoga class. I thought the exercise would help. I became friends with some of the people, and they invited me to join their meditation group. I can't believe how much better I feel about myself because I took the risk of joining."

PARADOX OF BLESSING AND CURSE

Because it is so painful, you consider your depression a curse. It is your thorn in the flesh that you beg God to remove. You may see yourself as a victim of your condition and ask, "Why me?" Your search for a cause only leads to dead ends. You may blame God, fate, your parents, or your defective mind. There is plenty of blame to throw around because you feel so targeted for misery and helpless to defend yourself. Cursing the day you were born with your condition only leads to an emotional hangover of apathy, anger, and bitterness.

Your depressed mind has tunnel vision, blind to the whole. Darkness dominates. It can only see the pain of endings and losses. However, your contemplative mind, bathed in sunlight and nourished with prayer and meditation, sees your condition differently. It views your life as a whole, from a larger perspective. It senses abundance, not scarcity. While not ignoring the suffering of loss, it also sees your depressive condition as a hidden blessing.

What is the blessing of sorrow? If you embrace it with loving acceptance, it can open your heart to compassion for others. Sadness and sorrow bring you to your knees. You learn your limits and gain humility. You discover your hidden attachments and learn to let go. The surrender opens up a life of new beginnings. It frees you to love wholeheartedly.

The suffering of depression can launch you on a spiritual path to growth and serenity. Confronted with the pain of loss, you have a choice about your relationship to it. You can reject it and become embittered. Or you can accept it, learn from it, and become compassionate toward others who suffer in a similar way. Many alcoholics end up thanking God for their condition because it allowed them to discover AA and turn their lives around. Seeing your condition also as a blessing can inspire gratitude and the generous desire to help others.

PRACTICE: CENTERING PRAYER

Father Thomas Keating, a Cistercian monk, developed a method of prayer to foster a contemplative attitude in your daily life. It is an attitude of being fully present in each moment of your life, aware of God's loving presence. His prayer method is called, "Centering Prayer," which opens your mind and heart to deepen your relationship with God (5). These are the guidelines for the prayer:

Choose a sacred word as a sign of your intention to surrender yourself to God's presence and action in your life. Spend some time in prayer and reflection to find a word that inspires you. It might be a word from Scripture, such as Father, Lord, Jesus, Mother Mary. It might be a word that expresses your highest aspirations, such as Love, Trust, Faith, Courage, Hope, Peace, or Let Go. Choose a word that has personal meaning for you, expressing your desire for communion with God.

Go to a quiet place where you will be alone. Sit comfortably with your eyes closed. Close your eyes to focus your attention on the stillness within you without outer distractions. Be relaxed, sitting with your back erect. Breathe deeply. Then, introduce your sacred word and repeat it to yourself slowly. Let the repetition help you focus on your center, where you sense God's loving presence.

Allow yourself to enter more deeply into the silence within you. Thoughts, feelings, sensations, and desires will inevitably arise. Do not fight them. Simply let them pass and keep your attention focused on the sacred word. During the prayer, even the sacred word may disappear. Gently let that pass also.

At the end of the prayer time, spend a few moments in silence. Sense that you are resting in God, and God is dwelling within you. Then, slowly open your eyes and resume your activities with an uplifted mind and heart and a sense of gratitude.

Spend at least 20 minutes in centering prayer. You can extend the time as you become more comfortable with the stillness and silence. Throughout the day during your normal activities, take a moment to center yourself and be fully present, as you were during the prayer time.

I add one word of caution. If you have been traumatized, an extended period of silence may be overwhelming for you because of the painful memories that may emerge from deep within your unconscious. Stop the practice if you are feeling overwhelmed. Return if and when you are ready.

With step eleven, you cultivate your relationship with God, your Higher Power, Ultimate Reality, through prayer and group involvement. Finding anchors in your life, you develop confidence to undertake your unique mission in life.

Dennis Ortman, Ph.D.

15

Share Life
Joyful Giving

Step Twelve: "Having had a spiritual awakening as a result of these Steps
we tried to carry this message to the depressed,
and to practice these principles in all our affairs."

"Don't ask what the world needs. Ask what makes you come alive, and go for it.
Because what the world needs is people who have come alive."

—Howard Thurman

As your journey continues, you surprise yourself that you feel more at home. You are adjusting to the darkness, as if you have night vision. You walk alertly and see the obstacles more clearly. The forest seems more alive with color, even in the fading light. You notice something you never noticed before. The woods are not silent. You hear birds, crickets, and night owls. You feel as if an inner light now guides you.

Step twelve expresses the third major theme of the Steps: "Help others." It encourages you to put into daily practice what you began in steps eight and nine, making amends and building relationships. Reaching out to others, the step promises, is the only path to a joyful life. The Steps/Traditions book states: "The joy of living is the theme of AA's twelfth step, and action is the key word. Here we turn outward toward our fellow alcoholics (sufferers) who are still in distress. Here we experience the kind of giving that asks no rewards" (p. 106).

JOYLESS INACTIVITY

Depression makes you shrink from life. Inwardly, you feel empty. Nothing gives you pleasure. Outwardly, you withdraw from life-giving activities. The result is joyless inactivity.

Ralph, a middle-aged man, came to see me after suffering a severe auto accident. He hobbled into my office using a walker and fell into a chair. He was obviously in pain. He began, "Doctor, I've been so depressed since the accident that I'm not sure I want to live. At first, I thanked God I survived, but now it seems like more of a curse than a blessing. I've been in so much pain. I push myself in physical therapy, but the progress is too slow. I'm impatient. And frankly, I'm discouraged that I'm ever going to get better."

It was obvious to me as I listened to his sad story that he had suffered a double loss. He lost both his physical health and his emotional wellbeing.

He continued, "I was always a confident man. I loved my job in construction and I kept myself physically active. I had so many hobbies—hunting, fishing, golf. Now I'm not sure if I'll ever be able to do any of those things again. The doctors won't give me a clear answer about my prognosis. I'm imagining I'll always be a cripple."

I sympathized with his loss and asked, "How do you cope?"

"I'm not sure I do," he said. "I just sit in my room and brood about things. My wife tries to encourage me and get me out as much as possible. But I just push her away, and anyone who tries to comfort me. I don't have any reason to live anymore like this. What is going to happen to me?"

Ralph was a man being consumed by his pain and his mood. The accident robbed him not only physically and emotionally, but also spiritually. He became dispirited. He was losing the will to live. In his desperation, Ralph was also a man ripe for a spiritual awakening.

AWAKENING A SLUMBERING SPIRIT

Recovery begins with an awakening of the spirit. What does it mean to have a spiritual awakening?

The Steps/Traditions book offers a helpful definition: "When a man or woman has a spiritual awakening, the most important meaning of it is that he has now become able to do, feel, and believe that which he could not do before on his unaided strength and resources alone. He has been granted a gift which amounts to a new state of consciousness and being" (p. 106-107). *Emotions Anonymous* adds: "Whatever form it may take, our awakening contains a characteristic attitude change. We have become less obsessed with our problems and pain and more open to other people" (p. 79).

The spiritual awakening is here described as, "a new state of consciousness," and, "an attitude change." Working the steps, you realized that such an awakening comes from both grace and effort. Some spiritual emergency, such as Ralph experienced, prepares the ground for a new blossoming of life. It creates a deep longing for something more to fill the void.

Albert Einstein famously remarked, "The significant problems we face cannot be solved on the same level of thinking we were at when we created them." What new kind of consciousness awakens for recovery? It is an awareness of life from a larger perspective, seeing loss, defeat, and dying as preludes to a new beginning. It involves a paradigm shift from scarcity to abundance thinking. Instead of believing yourself cursed by scarcity, you feel blessed by abundance, which leads to gratitude and generosity.

How does that new consciousness emerge?

THE GRIEVING-FORGIVING PROCESS

Anyone addicted to depression has fallen asleep. Some may awaken suddenly, in a dramatic fashion, like St. Paul who fell to the ground blinded and then saw in a new light. Most likely, you struggled with depression for a period of time until you finally admitted defeat. You wavered in finding strength in your faith. You also vacillated in recognizing and admitting the shortcomings your mood exposed. When you finally achieved a measure of peace, you suffered many relapses, as most addicts do. Even though awakened, you never felt completely secure in your recovery.

Recovery from depression demands letting go of the painful losses and the desire for revenge on those who harmed you. It is a process of coming to acceptance and forgiveness. Grieving and forgiving follow a similar path, with distinguishable moments and stages (1). Each stage presents its own challenges and contains seeds for new life.

DENIAL

Denial says, "It didn't happen." When the pain of loss is too much, you go into shock. For example, the loss of a loved one, a job, or a relationship may be overwhelming. You freeze up. Numb feelings and a foggy brain keep the pain at bay. The denial serves a purpose. It protects you from being overwhelmed. The lack of energy and interest in the world invites you to withdraw to nurse the wound. You become quiet and are alone with the pain until you are strong enough to address it directly.

Especially if you were traumatized by physical or sexual abuse as a child, you need to forget the pain to survive emotionally. The buried pain, however, lies dormant. It expresses itself indirectly through somatic complaints, dreams, blocked energy flow, and repeated self-defeating behavior. Your mood presents clues to the underlying pain. I have worked with patients who could only remember their abuse after years of therapy. One middle-aged woman came to me after being hypnotized at a party. Childhood memories of being sexually abused flooded her. These patients could only speak of the pain of betrayal when they were ready.

ANGER

You may break your silence with words of anger, screaming, "No!" You protest, "What happened to me should not have happened!" A sense of being wronged comes out. The injustice enrages you. Your anger may be expressed as blame with many targets—yourself, those who offended you, and cruel fate. The anger gives you a feeling of power that energizes you for constructive action. However, if it persists as resentment and bitterness, it may poison your life.

When the breakthrough of feelings occurs, some patients complain, "I feel like I have a volcano inside ready to explode. I must be getting worse." I tell them: "It's as if your hand was frostbitten. You don't feel pain and think everything is okay. But when your hand begins to thaw, you feel excruciating pain. You think you're getting worse. In reality, you are beginning to heal." The only way to heal is to go through the pain, with all the conflicting emotions, and not around it.

BARGAINING

"If only I had acted differently, then that terrible thing would not have happened," you tell yourself. Your bargaining mind speculates, "If only..." You create a fantasy world to avoid the pain. However, regret and guilt, if realistic, may awaken a sense of personal responsibility. You can learn from your mistakes. Often, we learn more from our failures than our successes.

You may discover that you bargain to avoid the pain of loss in many subtle ways. For example, you may persist in blaming others for your misery. You may engage in addictive behaviors to distract yourself or self-medicate the pain. You may continue to deny there is a problem. I tell my patients, "It's not the sadness and fear that harm you. Those feelings may be distressful, but they are not dangerous. It's all the ways you've devised to avoid the pain that cause real harm. They restrict you and choke off your life."

DEPRESSION

At some point, the sadness and sorrow will hit you with full force. You will realize the full extent of the loss you suffered. You cannot avoid facing the pain. The emptiness is inescapable. Your depressed mind laments, "I can't tolerate the loss!" The hurt exposes your tender spots, your vulnerability, what you cannot imagine living without. As uncomfortable as it is, however, allowing yourself to feel the pain is essential to your healing. You learn that the pain cannot defeat you because you survive it. You are bruised, but not broken.

Depression plants seeds of compassion in your heart. Suffering opens your heart to the suffering of others. It creates empathy for their vulnerability and the desire to relieve your own and others' suffering. Being aware of your sadness, you learn about your sensitivities and begin to reflect on how you need to care for yourself.

ACCEPTANCE

Acceptance proclaims, "Yes" to life. Instead of hanging on to the memory of your past wounds and your fixed ideas about how your life should have been, you embrace your present experience. Instead of nurturing anger against those who harmed you, you extend the hand of forgiveness. Most importantly, you hold yourself with unconditional friendliness, despite your faults and failings. You accept your current life wholeheartedly as it is, not as you wish it would be. You can embrace life's challenges because you see the big picture. All the endings announce new beginnings. Hope springs eternal. This is the long-awaited fruit of spiritual awakening from working the steps.

Acceptance opens your heart and mind to newness. You have faith you can survive and grow from further pain. You have hope you can move on and build a new life. Your broken heart enables you to love more intimately with a compassionate heart. With renewed strength and courage, you are able to adjust to the inevitable changes in life. As the Sufi mystic Rumi advised, "Don't grieve. Anything you lose comes around in another form."

Joel, awakened by his depression:

"Growing up, I felt like a loser. My father was alcoholic, and he always picked on me. I joined a motorcycle club when I was in my twenties, probably just to piss him off. I was married at the time and had a child, but I didn't care about my responsibilities then. I was drinking heavily and felt like I belonged with the club. I saw myself as a loser and joined a group of losers. At first I really enjoyed it. People feared us whenever we went into the bars. I felt powerful, like a somebody. Many in the group got drunk and started fights. Of course, because we were a brotherhood, we all jumped into the fray.

After a while, the lifestyle began to wear on me. I think I was depressed, but didn't know it. My wife complained about me being away all the time, but I just ignored her. I knew that all the violence wasn't really me. After one big bar fight, I became physically sick. I thought about suicide and took an overdose of pills. I was admitted to a psychiatric hospital where I was diagnosed with depression and prescribed medication. That was a turning point in my life. I stopped drinking, went to AA meetings, and got a regular job. I realized how much I neglected my family. Listening to my depression saved my life."

Working through your depression, taking seriously its message, you awaken your true self. Your dark mood covers you like a blanket. Lifting the mood releases the energy of your inner spirit. It is a spirit of wisdom that sees life as it is, of compassion that seeks to relieve suffering, and of mercy that accepts all.

GRATEFULLY LIVING LARGER

The awakening of your spirit creates a new mind and heart. Your new consciousness is one of abundance that naturally expresses itself in gratitude, joy, and generosity. You see life as a precious gift and want to share what you received. Your light has been hidden under a dark blanket. Now you desire to show it.

How do you use the awakened energy? How do you show your light?

HELPING FELLOW SUFFERERS

After Bill Wilson "got religion," he became sober and began to turn his life around. He looked for a way to have "a quality sobriety" without the emotional hangovers of resentment, pettiness, and fear. He met with other struggling alcoholics and formulated the Twelve Steps for recovery, based on his personal experience and research on spiritual traditions. He believed that alcoholics could understand each other in ways that no one else could. They shared an experience with alcohol that bonded them. He created a fellowship, a place for alcoholics to meet and support each other. A key to recovery, he discovered, was overcoming the self-centeredness that spawned the addiction.

Helping others was the way out.

Caught up in depression, you can understand a fellow sufferer like no one else. While others may stigmatize and become impatient with depressed people, you have empathy.

You understand. You can be a blessing to others who share your affliction. Sharing what you learn in your recovery can help set them free. It will also bring you joy and further your own recovery.

You have a wonderful gift to give that can help relieve the suffering of many.

WIDENING THE CIRCLE OF CARE

With whom do you share this gift? How do you practice these principles in all your affairs? You begin, of course, with yourself. When I suggest the importance of self-care to some of my patients, they object, "That is selfish."

"Is it okay to be good to yourself?" I ask.

"That's alright. It sounds better," they respond.

Then, I proceed to explore their reluctance to care for themselves. "I don't believe I'm worth it. Besides, I was taught it is better to care for others," they say.

"But if you don't care for yourself, how can you care for others?" I ask. "Consider the love commandment. Jesus said to love your neighbor as yourself. The important word is 'as.' He did not say love your neighbor 'more' than yourself or 'less' than yourself. He said to love equally. The trick is to keep a balance between loving others and loving yourself. Or to put it another way, to recognize your oneness with others and love them as another self."

Drunk with sadness, you may not know how to take care of yourself. Preoccupied with the pain and getting rid of it, you become disconnected from yourself, out of touch with your needs. It requires a concerted effort to stop, look, and pay attention to your desires. When you know what is important to you, you can then muster the motivation to do something about it.

Jeremy, ambitious for himself:

"I'm in college, but I'm failing. My parents are on my case. I just don't care about all the classes. They don't interest me, and I don't see how I can use them. That's made me depressed. I've been thinking about what I really like. I love computers and making video games. My friends and I are working on a game we'd like to sell. When I'm working on the game and thinking about it, I feel alive. My mood lifts. I came to realize that the opposite of depression is ambition, even if my ambition is not the same as my parents."

Your second outreach is to those who are in your circle of intimacy, your partner, family, and friends. How can you extend yourself to them? A popular book by Gary Chapman, entitled, *The 5 Love Languages* (2), suggests practical ways of improving intimate relationships. He suggests that everyone has their own natural way of giving and receiving love that makes them feel connected. The five love languages are: 1) words of affirmation; 2) quality time; 3) receiving gifts; 4) acts of service; 5) physical touch. These different languages are self-explanatory. However, you need to pay close attention to how you naturally give and prefer to receive love in relationships. Notice also the preferred style of giving and receiving of the significant people in your life. Matching your love languages promises to give you a sense of closeness and to overcome your depressed isolation.

All the religious traditions remind us that we are members of a larger body. They call us to serve others beyond our immediate family. These traditions provide concrete suggestions on how to implement the commandment to love one another. For example, the works of mercy from the Catholic tradition suggest practical ways of helping others:

Corporal works of mercy:

- feeding the hungry.
- giving drink to the thirsty.
- clothing the naked.
- sheltering the homeless.
- visiting the sick.
- ransoming the captive.
- burying the dead.

Spiritual works of mercy:

- instructing the ignorant.
- counseling the doubtful.
- admonishing the sinner.
- bearing wrongs patiently.
- forgiving offenses.
- comforting the afflicted.
- praying for the living and the dead.

Life is difficult. Many opportunities are presented for you to show kindness and compassion, if you are aware and willing.

Your depressed mind thinks small, mostly about yourself. Your enlarged consciousness embraces the world, acknowledging your connection with all beings. For example, the Hindu myth of Indra's net expresses the interconnectedness of all. The god Indra hangs a net over his palace at the axis of the world, which reaches without limit in all directions. A single glittering jewel hangs from each of the countless nodes of the net. The jewels shine like stars in the firmament. If you closely inspect an individual jewel, you discover that it reflects all the other jewels in the net, infinite in number. And each jewel reflected in this one jewel reflects all the other jewels, creating an infinite mirroring process.

All beings, animate and inanimate, are jewels in the universe's net, reflecting each other's beauty. Our care extends not only to all human beings, but to our entire planet. With our current ecological crisis and diminishing resources, we are called to a global consciousness. Natural disasters across the world impact everyone on this spaceship Earth. Starvation, plagues, and violence, even on another continent, immediately affect us. Consequently, we feel a sense of responsibility to use our resources wisely, to care for our environment, and to live in harmony with nature. We have a shared destiny on this tiny planet in a vast universe. Seeing yourself as an essential part of this near infinite whole affirms both your smallness and greatness.

How are you, as an individual, to contribute? You have a unique calling, a gift that only you can give to the universe. Your life task is to discover that gift and share it. A story by the Persian poet Rumi expresses the uniqueness of your vocation: "A King sent you to a country to carry out one special, specific task. You go to the country and you perform a hundred other tasks, but if you have not performed the task you were sent for, it is as if you have performed nothing at all. So man has come into the world for a particular task and that is his purpose. If he doesn't perform it, he will have done nothing" (3).

Your joy will come from discovering and living your life task. That calling is your personal way of helping others. For example, you may feel called to serve the poor, write a book, or work on family relationships. Your depression suggests that you have lost yourself and your mission in life. The pain propels you to explore deeply what is missing and what deeper longings are seeking expression. Just pay attention. Listen to the message of your mood.

UNDEFEATED BY DEPRESSION
LINCOLN AND MOTHER TERESA

You are not alone in your depression. Many people who have made significant contributions to improving the world suffered severe depression. The mood did not defeat them. Instead, it sensitized them to pursue their unique missions in life. Two models for me are Abraham Lincoln and Mother Teresa.

Abraham Lincoln suffered bouts of depression throughout his life (4). As a young man, he had suicidal thoughts, and his family watched him closely so he would not harm himself. He certainly suffered many personal losses that took a toll on him, his mother, his beloved sister, and his sons. He felt deeply the pain of the nation in the throes of a civil war and a sense of responsibility for the deaths of so many. His law partner observed, "His melancholy dripped from him as he walked." Lincoln, an extremely private person, said of himself, "I am now the most miserable man living. If what I felt were distributed to the whole human family there would be not one happy face on the earth. I must die or be better it appears to me."

This sensitive, thoughtful, melancholic man carried the weight of the nation on his shoulders. He lived with a profound sense of the tragic in life. His depression opened his heart to the suffering of his people. Compassion moved him to push for reform to relieve their suffering. As president, he gained a sense of vital purpose that transcended his moods. He refused to be controlled by his moods and dedicated himself to his dual agenda, to preserve the union and stop the spread of slavery. Aware of the grace of God in his life, his undaunted efforts transformed his personal suffering into a gateway to his greatness.

Agnes Bohaxhiu, an Albanian girl, knew at a young age that she was called to devote her life to the service of God. She joined the Loreto Sisters and took the name Sister Mary Teresa of the Child Jesus. Her life appeared to be moving in one direction, until it was suddenly interrupted on a dusty train ride in India. She received what she identified as, "a call within a call," from God to establish a new religious order. She related that the message from God was clear, "I was to leave the convent and help the poor while living among them. It was an order. To fail it would have been to break faith." She fought patiently and persistently with Church authorities to found her order, the Missionary Sisters of Charity, dedicated to serving "the poorest of the poor."

The accomplishments of this dedicated, faith-filled, humble person are obvious. However, what were not so well known were her inner struggles, which were revealed with the publication of her letters to her spiritual director (5). For nearly fifty years she felt unloved and unwanted by God, writing, "The place of God in my soul is blank. There is no God in me." She felt no emotional or spiritual consolations from her faith. Some believed she suffered a loss of faith or clinical depression. But they were wrong.

Mother Teresa persisted in her prayer and work despite spiritual and emotional dryness. What she experienced was, "a dark night of the spirit" that purified her faith. Instead of giving up in despair, she found meaning in her experience of darkness. She wrote, "If I ever become a saint, I will surely be one of 'darkness.' I will continually be absent from Heaven—to light the light of those in darkness on Earth." She identified with the suffering of Jesus on the cross and with the plight of the poor she served. Her empty feelings and longings motivated her to work more selflessly.

Your depression is "a dark night of the emotions." It is similar to a dark night of the spirit. Your depressive dark night purifies your motivations and calls you to maturity. The pain moves you to give up the emotional clinging caused by your belief that you cannot be happy without particular persons and things in your life.

The list of those who have made great contributions by transforming their moods into a vital purpose is long: Winston Churchill, Teddy, Franklin, and Eleanor Roosevelt, Edgar Allan Poe, Vincent Van Gogh, Pyotr Tchaikovsky, Lord Byron, and so forth. Their depression inspired enormous creativity and purpose in their lives. They refused to be victims of their moods. Read their biographies, reflect on their strength in adversity, and learn from them.

PARADOX OF GIVING AND RECEIVING

In a depressed state of mind, you live with a clenched fist. Preoccupied with all you have lost, you are terrified of losing more. What do you fear losing? The list is endless: your health, a loved one, your possessions, your good image, and so forth. You entertain the belief that if you hang on tightly enough you will be secure. You also imagine that if you give up something, it is lost forever. Your depressed mind follows a zero-balance way of thinking. There is only a limited supply of whatever you desire, and once it is used up, it is gone.

The twelfth step of recovery insists on turning away from yourself to help others. The step confronts you with a paradox: "We give it away to keep it." That statement confounds the logic of your depressed mind. It also challenges your self-centered urge to protect yourself at all costs and to open your hands to others. The paradox echoes the wisdom of the *Tao Te Ching*:

**Serve the needs of others,
And all your needs will be fulfilled.
Through selfless action, fulfillment is attained (7).**

How is that possible? Look around you with your enlarged consciousness. The earth continually gives without asking in return. It only invites you to participate in its ongoing cycle of renewal. The air you breathe, the food you eat, the water you drink, and the sunshine that warms you comes from the abundance of the earth. That abundance comes from a hidden, eternal Source we may call God, Ultimate Reality, or the Life Force.

Gratitude for what you receive inspires your generosity. You give because you recognize you have already received so much more. I begin each day at work with an aspiration from an unknown source: "As the earth gives us food and air and all the things we need, may I give my heart to caring for all others until all attain awakening. For the good of all sentient beings, may loving kindness be born in me." I pray that this intention guides my interactions with my patients.

Trust also your own experience, rather than your biased mind. When you give yourself wholeheartedly in love, without expecting anything in return, the rewards are astonishing. You feel an inner joy and peace. Often, by the law of attraction, the person who receives your love responds with love. It creates a bond of intimacy between you and the person. Even if you do not receive appreciation or gratitude, you know in your heart you were true to yourself. In being yourself, you experience great joy and freedom.

PRACTICE: THE FIVE REMEMBRANCES

In your depression, you feel tossed about by the winds of change. Change is your enemy because it creates losses. You long for something permanent, reliable, and predictable. You look for some solid ground on which to stand firm.

The Buddha taught his followers that happiness comes only from accepting the facts of life. The most basic fact is that change is constant. Everything is impermanent, in constant flux. However, he taught them that one thing lasts, their actions and their ongoing consequences. To help them accept the truth of impermanence, he invited them to meditate regularly on what are called "the five remembrances."

1) I am of the nature to grow old. There is no way to escape growing old.

2) I am of the nature to have ill health. There is no way to escape ill health.

3) I am of the nature to die. There is no way to escape death.

4) All that is dear to me and everyone I love are of the nature to change. There is no way to escape being separated from them.

5) My actions are my only true belongings. I cannot escape the consequences of my actions. My actions are the ground upon which I stand.

Take some time each day to reflect on these five facts of life. Your immediate reaction may be that these remembrances are depressing and will only bring you down. But think more carefully. They express fundamental truths of your experience about aging, health, change, and death. Accepting these facts of life can help you change your perspective and appreciate the wonder of your life. They remind you to live the present moment fully. Your time is precious because it is so limited. Despite all the changing circumstances of your life, you still have freedom to choose how you want to act.

Your actions, over which you have control, are the firm ground on which you stand.

The practice of the five remembrances concretizes the Serenity Prayer, distinguishing what you can and cannot change. You can only change your own behavior, which affects your destiny. Embracing the complexity of your life, you gain serenity, courage, and wisdom.

The first eleven steps culminate in the twelfth step, a call to action. Your spiritual awakening loosened the bond of your depressed mood, freeing you to pursue what you value most in life. Living your unique life task and serving others are the keys to finding joy and fulfillment.

Epilogue
The Journey Is Home

"Each day is the journey and the journey itself is home."

—Basho

"Just when the caterpillar thought the world was over,
it became a butterfly."

—Anonymous

You began this journey into the dark forest with a goal in mind. You wanted to get through it and survive. Wandering the tortuous path, you hoped to find a rainbow at the end. You believed you were going somewhere better. Now your mood and expectations are changing with the changing light. The shadows, especially your own, do not frighten you so much. You do not run away in fear. The dawning atmosphere, with brief bright spots, provides enough comfort. Besides, an inner light guides your way. You actually enjoy the colorful woods and sounds of life. You tell yourself, "I'm at home here."

LAURA'S STORY CONTINUED

Laura continued to be stuck in her depressed mood. Nothing excited her. She accommodated her family by continuing to take her medications and to see her psychologist. During sessions, she was mostly quiet or complained about how little interest she had in living. During one session, the therapist asked her, "What would you do if you weren't depressed?"

"I don't know. I don't want to do anything but sleep," she said.

"What did you do before you were depressed?" he persisted.

"I took care of the family. I cleaned, cooked, and made sure everyone was happy," she responded.

"Did you enjoy doing those things?" the doctor inquired.

"I did then, but I don't want to do those things now," she replied.

"What changed?"

"I got cancer and lost my mother," she said.

The doctor knew from her history that she had been a caretaker from childhood. She attended to everyone's needs but her own and likely lost herself. She had become submissive and never asserted herself. The doctor suspected that her depressed mood disguised her resentment at all the demands made on her and her desire to assert herself. He offered her an interpretation. "Perhaps your depressed mood is a protest against all the demands made on you to take care of everyone. Now you want to find some way to care for yourself and do what you really want to do." Laura listened, but remained quiet. The doctor continued, "I'd like you to try going to a support group. You don't have to go unless you want to. It's only a suggestion because I think it would help. You don't even have to talk at the group unless you want to. Just listen and see what you learn about yourself."

Laura thought for a moment and said, "Okay, I'll try it."

Because Laura did not want to go alone, her sister, who also suffered bouts of depression, agreed to accompany her. Both entered the room marked, "Emotions Anonymous Meeting," with trepidation. Laura felt the tension drain from her with the warm welcome of the group leader and all the other members. As each member shared their emotional struggles in the table discussion, Laura paid close attention and began to see herself in them. The ideas about being powerless over your emotions and the uselessness of self-hatred resonated with her. Laura did not speak, but she listened. She sensed a crack in her wall of depression. She told her sister after the meeting, "I think I'll come back next week."

A PILGRIM'S PROGRESS

Your life journey may take you, for a time, into a dark forest. Actually, because being alive means changing, and changing often, you will frequently feel the pain of loss and longing for new life. How do you adjust to the constant flux of your life? You have a choice. You can be a nomad, a chameleon, or a pilgrim, as this poem of unknown origin suggests (1): (quoted in Lepo)

To journey without being changed
is to be a nomad.
To change without journeying
is to be a chameleon.
To journey and to be transformed
by the journey
is to be a pilgrim.

When stuck in a depressed mood, you wander through life like a nomad or chameleon. You have a sense of homelessness, not belonging. You resist the challenges of changes imposed on you against your will. Overwhelmed by a sense of loss and your own scarcity thinking, you cling to fixed ideas about how your life should be, or you refuse to assert yourself in pursuing your goals and sleepwalk through life. At the heart of your depressed mood is the fantasy of control. You want your life to be just the way you want it.

In choosing to be a pilgrim, however, you have decided to embrace and learn from all the losses change brings. You become fully engaged in your life journey without trying to escape any challenges that arise. You embrace completely your experience in the moment without withdrawing into your fixed ideas. You accept your current life, with all its joys and sorrows, as the place of your happiness and wellbeing. It is here, not there, that you discover your true self. It is now, not then, that you find contentment.

As a pilgrim, you live the paradox that your journey is your home and your home is your journey. You need not look outside yourself and your life to find your truth. You are restless, searching, and willing to be surprised. Receptive to the new, you discover the wonder and mystery of life. You recognize your essential connection with the entire universe, everyone and everything. Your deepest longings for the Infinite, the Eternal, the Still Point are fulfilled in the here and now. It is the treasure already there for the taking. Abundance surrounds you. As T.S. Eliot expressed it (2):

We shall not cease from exploration
And the end of all our exploring
Will be to arrive where we started
And know the place for the first time.

THE BIG QUESTIONS

The pain of your depression launches you on your search. The steps are your guide. What are you looking for during your journey? The poet Rainer Marie Rilke advises, "Be patient toward all that is unsolved in your heart and try to love the questions themselves." Four big questions emerge that cry out for exploring more than answering. These questions are particularly urgent when you are depressed because you have lost yourself, your meaning in life, and your way.

WHO AM I?

Your depressed brain is sensitive to loss. Because you are alive, you experience constant changes, which involve losses and potential gains. Only the dead are static. However, your depressed mind cannot tolerate continual cycles of change with all their uncertainty. To compensate, you fixate your thinking and reacting. Your mind stews about the past and all the pain of losses suffered. You withdraw from the flow of life, seeking an island of safety in inactivity. In the process, you assume a fixed identity as a "depressed person." Ironically, while seeking to be alive, you become dead with your static thinking and behaving.

But you are discovering another way. The pain of self-doubt and confusion can motivate you to become a pilgrim on a journey to uncover your true self. It propels you on a personal search. Your identity is not so fixed, static, and frozen. In reality, you are a mystery that participates in the Divine. In being consciously aware, you experience your own depth, freedom, and creativity. Like a pilgrim, you search with an open mind and heart to discover your own depth, richness, and uniqueness. Attentive to the flow of your experience, you see many changing aspects of yourself and are open to the surprise of discovery. You are in wonder and awe of yourself as a reflection of the Mystery of God.

WHERE DID I COME FROM?

Depression creates emotional, mental, and spiritual amnesia. You may not remember ever being happy or lose hope you will ever be happy again. You feel lost, not knowing who you are, where you came from, or where you are going. The past and future are absorbed in a pain-filled present. You live in a trance of forgetfulness of the love and nurturing you receive from your parents, friends, and family. You ignore the blessings of the good earth and the support of the community.

Alone and lost, you wander like a person in a desert dying of thirst and searching for some oasis. You may see yourself born under a curse. Bad genes and bad luck control your life. Depression is your fate, and there is nothing you can do about it.

Your thirst and desire for life, however, can drive you to seek your roots. Where did you ultimately come from? You seek some wellspring of life and nourishment. Your thirst can awaken your mind of abundance, which sees more clearly what is present around and within you. You awaken from your slumber to remember and reconnect with life and its Source, the Divine.

Your mood makes you a natural contemplative. In meditating on your situation, you wake up to how much your life is a precious gift, sustained by the abundance of the earth and the love of many. You recognize the inexhaustible Source from which everything arises and returns. It brings spring flowers, rebirth, and new relationships. You drink from that wellspring and come alive. As your heart opens, gratitude replaces resentment, generosity overcomes greed, and hope springs from despair. The *Tao Te Ching* expresses further consequences of this discovery in your life:

> **Returning to the source is serenity.**
> **If you don't realize the source,**
> **you stumble in confusion and sorrow.**
> **When you realize where you come from,**
> **you naturally become tolerant,**
> **disinterested, amused,**
> **kindhearted as a grandmother,**
> **dignified as a king (16).**

WHY AM I HERE?

"To be or not to be?" Hamlet asks. Severe depression makes the question urgent, a matter of life or death. Camus, the French existentialist writer said, "There is but one truly serious philosophical problem, and that is suicide. Judging whether life is or is not worth living amounts to answering the fundamental question of philosophy." You became depressed because what you deemed necessary for your happiness was taken away. The death of a loved one, a lost job, or a change in health can turn your world upside down. Then, you search for the meaning of your life in the face of the loss. What can replace it? How can you imagine life without it? Finding the meaning within the loss will determine whether you live in hope or despair. It will determine whether you want to live or die.

Suffering loss interrupts the flow of your life. It creates a crisis. Your old security, satisfaction, and sense of purpose are upset. The disruption can motivate you to seek a deeper meaning in your life and to make a choice. Will you cling to the past or accept the new life the future offers? Can the lost love open your heart to love again more deeply? Can the lost job propel you into a new, more satisfying career? Can your decline in health make you more compassionate? In the process of grieving, you loosen your emotional bond to what you loved so you can love again—in a new way. You explore what you really value, what can last in the ongoing changes of life. You look for what will make your life worth living, embracing your unique life task.

WHERE AM I GOING?

Captivated by a mood, you feel imprisoned in your life. That prison can become a familiar place, not really comfortable, but secure. You can avoid a life that appears more threatening to you. Where do you want to go? When you are addicted to depression, you do not want to go anywhere. You only want to hide behind the safe walls of your mood and sleep your life away. Or you may want to escape into some world of fantasy, some imagined heaven. Or worse, escape by suicide.

Your dark mood, of course, is also a protest against your life as it is. You want more. Most likely, the way you are living does not match who you are as a person. It may be that the way you are spending your precious time and energy is worthless compared to your gifts and values. If you ignore your talents and skills, others are deprived of what you can offer. You hold the key to your self-created prison. Releasing yourself embarks you on a journey of self-discovery of what is important for you in life. Your values and talents become the guideposts on your journey. They tell you where you want to go.

THE JOY OF BEING YOURSELF

As a pilgrim, you feel free to explore your life in the here and now. There is no other life. This is it. As you discover your values and skills, you are faced with a choice. You can let your fluctuating moods control you, or you can choose to live according to your values and share your gifts.

When I ask my patients about their goals in life, many tell me, "I want to be happy."

"What keeps you from being happy?" I ask.

"My depression," they say. "If I only were not depressed, I would be a happy person."

"You give your mood a lot of power!" I say, and then explain: "Seeking happiness is like chasing the wind. If you try to grasp it, it slips through your fingers. Happiness is the byproduct of living the life you're meant to live. When you are simply yourself, living your own life, you discover you are content. Your real life task is to find your true self and let your light shine." You find joy in giving yourself away and not clinging to yourself. Many of my depressed patients have told me that their spirits were lifted by visiting sick friends in the hospital. They forgot about their pain for a moment, showed compassion, and found joy.

PARADOX OF SORROW AND JOY

In the throes of a depressive episode, you naturally want to eliminate all sorrow from your life. You long for the joy that eludes you. Because you have felt so overwhelmed by the pain of loss, you fantasize about a world without suffering, with only bliss. You long for heaven on earth.

Your natural instinct to avoid the pain, however, disengages you from life as it is. Your fantasy of a perfect world is really a death wish. What you desire is a world without change, a static existence. There is no movement, or life, because you are then fixed in one permanent state of imagined joy.

The world of the here and now is a world in constant flux. It moves, changes, transforms. It is alive. Change, which can be unpleasant, is a sign of life. New life emerges through an often painful process of dying. Endings announce new beginnings. Losses prepare for gains. Embracing the whole cycle of life opens you to the experience of both sorrow and joy. You cannot have one without the other. Sorrow contains the seeds of joy, while joy anticipates sorrow. Accepting the inevitable sorrows of life enriches and deepens your experience. It makes you a compassionate person who can also appreciate the joy of being alive. As the Chinese proverb states, "Who has never tasted what is bitter does not know what is sweet."

On your pilgrimage, you are responsible for yourself, but do not travel alone. The path is perilous. You need all the like-minded company you can get. The journey home to yourself, becoming aware of your connection to a larger whole, has many twists and turns. You face numerous obstacles within yourself, especially your fears and moods and addictive thinking. Trusting in your Higher Power, you can welcome all the inevitable challenges and face them with courage and determination. Grace envelops you. You can proceed with hope, confident that you will arrive at your destination if you persevere.

Endnotes

Introduction

1. R. Kessler, P. Berglund, O. Demler, et al., (2005). "Lifetime prevalence of age-of-on-set distribution of DSM-IV disorder in the National Comorbidity Survey Replication," *Archives of General Psychiatry* no 63 (2005): 593-602. K. Merikangas, J. He, M. Burstein, et al., (2010). "Lifetime prevalence of mental disorders in U.S. adolescents: Results from the National Comorbidity Survey Replication—Adolescent Supplement (NCS-A)," *Journal of the American Academy of Child and Adolescent Psychiatry* no 49 (2010): 980-989.

2. Stephen Iliardi, *The Depression Cure: The 6-Step Program to Beat Depression without Drugs*

3. (Cambridge: Da Capo Press, 2010), 41.

4. All quotes from the *Tao Te Ching* are from Stephen Mitchell's translation, *Tao Te Ching* (New York: Harper Perennial Classics, 2000).

Chapter One

1. D. Regier, M. Farmer, D. Rae, et al., "Comorbidity of mental disorders with alcohol and other drug abuse. Results from the Epidemiologic Catchment Area (ECA) Study," *Journal of the American Medical Association* no 264 (1995): 2511-2528.

Chapter Three

1. Paul Gilbert, *Overcoming Depression: A Self-Help Guide Using Cognitive Behavioral Techniques* (New York: Basic Books, 1977), 16-26.

2. Iliardi, viii.

Chapter Four

1. All the Steps/Traditions quotes are from *Twelve Steps and Twelve Traditions* (New York: Alcoholics Anonymous World Services, Inc., 2012).

2. All the Big Book quotes are from *Alcoholics Anonymous: The Big Book*, fourth edition (New York: Alcoholics Anonymous World Services, Inc., 2001).

Chapter Five

1. All the Emotions Anonymous quotes are from *Emotions Anonymous*, revised edition (Saint Paul: Emotions Anonymous International Services, 1994).

Chapter Six

1. Stephen Iliardi, *The Depression Cure: The 6-Step Program to Beat Depression without Drugs* (Cambridge: Da Capo Press, 2010). Gabriel Cousens, *Depression-Free for Life: A Physician's All-Natural, 5-Step Plan* (New York: HarperCollins, 2000).

2. Jon Kabat-Zinn, *Full Catastrophe Living* (New York: Bantam Books, 2013), 75-97.

Chapter Seven

1. Diana Butler Bass, *Christianity after Religion: The End of Church and the Birth of a New Spiritual Awakening* (New York: HarperOne, 2012), 46.

2. Bass, 76-83.

3. "Four Quartets: Burnt Norton," in T.S. Eliot, *Collected Poems: 1909-1962* (London: Faber and Faber, 1974).

4. T.S. Eliot, "Four Quartets: East Coker."

5. Jon Kabat-Zinn, 54-74.

Chapter Eight

1. *Twelve Steps and Twelve Traditions*, 34, 40.

2. T.S. Eliot, "Four Quartets: The Dry Salvages."

3. 2008 Pew Study as reported in Bass, 49.

4. Reported in Bass, 49.

5. *Alcoholics Anonymous: The Big Book*, 12.

6. Joseph Goldstein, *Insight Meditation* (Boston: Shambhala, 2003).

Chapter Nine

1. *Twelve Steps and Twelve Traditions*, 42.

2. All Bible quotes are from *The New American Bible* (New Jersey: Thomas Nelson, 1971).

3. Thomas Keating, *The Heart of the World* (New York: Crossroad Publishing Company), 47-55.

Chapter Ten

1. Coleman Barks, *The Essential Rumi* (London: Penguin, 2004), 109.

2. Sharon Salzburg, *Loving-Kindness* (Boston: Shambhala, 2002).

Chapter Eleven

1. T.S. Eliot, "Four Quartets: Burnt Norton."

Chapter Twelve

1. Steven Hayes, *Get out of Your Mind and into Your Life: The New Acceptance and Commitment Therapy* (Oakland: New Harbinger, 2005), 170-176.

2. *Twelve Steps and Twelve Traditions*, 83.

3. Pema, Chodron, *The Places that Scare You* (Boston: Shambhala, 2001), 55-60.

Chapter Thirteen

1. Quoted in Richard Rohr, *Breathing Under Water* (Cincinnati: St. Anthony Messenger Press, 2011), 103.

2. Shantideva, *The Way of the Bodhisattva*, trans. Padmakara Translation Group (Boston: Shambhala, 1997), verse 48.

3. Gregg Krech, *Naikan: Gratitude, Grace, and the Japanese Art of Self-Reflection* (Berkeley: Stone Bridge Press, 2002).

Chapter Fourteen

1. Thich Nhat Hanh, *Being Peace* (Berkeley: Parallax Press, 1987), 15.

2. Thomas Merton, *New Seeds of Contemplation* (New York: New Directions Publ., 1972), 36.

3. *Alcoholics Anonymous: The Big Book*, 17.

4. Bass, 39-71.

5. Keating, Thomas, *Open Mind, Open Heart* (New York: Bloomsbury, 2006).

Chapter Fifteen

1. Elizabeth Kubler-Ross, *On Death and Dying* (New York: Scribner, 1969).

2. Gary Chapman, *The 5 Love Languages: The Secret to Love That Lasts* (Chicago: Northfield Publishing, 1992).

3. Quoted in James Hollis, *Finding Meaning in the Second Half of Life* (New York: Gotham), 102.

4. Joshua Wolf Shenk, *Lincoln's Melancholy: How Depression Challenged a President and Fueled His Greatness* (New York: Mariner Books, 2006).

5. Mother Teresa, *Come Be My Light: The Private Writings of the "Saint of Calcutta."* Ed. Brian Kolodiejchuk. (New York: Doubleday, 2007).

Epilogue

1. As quoted in Mark Lepo, *The Book of Awakening* (San Francisco: Conari Press), 34.

2. T.S. Eliot, "Four Quartets: Little Gidding."

Dennis Ortman, Ph.D.

Suggested Readings

Alcoholics Anonymous: The Big Book. Fourth edition. New York: Alcoholics Anonymous World Services, Inc., 2001.

Alexander, William. *Ordinary Recovery: Mindfulness, Addiction, and the Path of Lifelong Sobriety*. Boston: Shambhala, 2010.

Bass, Diana Butler. *Christianity after Religion: The End of Church and the Birth of a New Spiritual Awakening*. New York: HarperOne, 2012.

Bien, Thomas, and Bien, Beverly. *Mindful Recovery: A Spiritual Path to Healing from Addiction*. New York: John Wiley and Sons, 2002.

Brach, Tara. *Radical Acceptance: Embracing Your Life with the Heart of a Buddha*. New York: Bantam Book, 2003.

Chapman, Gary. *The 5 Love Languages: The Secret to Love That Lasts*. Chicago: Northfield Publishing, 1992.

Chodron, Pema. *The Places that Scare You*. Boston: Shambhala, 2001.

Cousens, Gabriel. *Depression-Free for Life: A Physician's All-Natural, 5-Step Plan*. New York: HarperCollins, 2000).

Dodd, Lance. *The Heart of Addiction*. New York: Harper-Collins, 2002.

Eliot, T.S. *Collected Poems: 1909-1962*. London: Faber and Faber, 1974.

Emotions Anonymous. Revised edition. Saint Paul: Emotions Anonymous International Services, 1994.

Germer, Christopher. *The Mindful Path to Self-Compassion: Freeing Yourself from Destructive Thoughts and Emotions*. New York: Guilford Press, 2009.

Gilbert, Paul. *Overcoming Depression: A Self-Help Guide Using Cognitive Behavioral Techniques.*, New York: Basic Books, 1977.

Goldstein, Joseph. *Insight Meditation: The Practice of Freedom*. Boston: Shambhala, 2003.

Griffin, Kevin. *One Breath at a Time: Buddhism and the Twelve Steps.* New York: St. Martin's Press, 2004.

Grof, Christina. *The Thirst for Wholeness: Attachment, Addiction, and the Spiritual Path.* New York: HarperCollins, 1993.

Hayes, Steven. *Get out of Your Mind and into Your Life: The New Acceptance and Commitment Therapy.,* Oakland: New Harbinger, 2005.

Hollis, James. *Creating a Life: Finding Your Individual Path.* Toronto: Inner City Books, 2001.

Hollis, James. *Finding Meaning in the Second Half of Life: How to Finally, Really Grow Up.* New York: Gotham Books, 2005.

Hollis, James. *What Matters Most: Living a More Considered Life.* New York: Gotham Books, 2009.

Hollis, James. *Hauntings: Dispelling the Ghosts Who Run Our Lives.* Ashville: Chiron Publications, 2013.

Honos-Webb, Lara. *Listening to Depression: How Understanding Your Pain Can Heal Your Life.* Oakland: New Harbinger, 2006.

Iliardi, Stephen. *The Depression Cure: The 6-Step Program to Beat Depression without Drugs.* Cambridge: Da Capo Press, 2010.

Jacobs-Stewart, Therese. *Mindfulness and the 12 Steps: Living recovery in the present moment.* Center City: Hazelden, 2010.

Jamison, Kay Redfield. *An Unquiet Mind: A Memoir of Moods and Madness.* New York: Vintage Books, 1996.

Kabat-Zinn, Jon. *Full Catastrophe Living.* New York: Bantam Books, 2013.

Keating, Thomas. *Open Mind, Open Heart.* New York: Bloomsbury, 2006.

Keating, Thomas. *The Heart of the World: An Introduction to Contemplative Christianity.* New York: Crossroad Publishing Company, 2008.

Keating, Thomas. *Divine Therapy and Addiction: Centering Prayer and the Twelve Steps.* New York: Lantern Books, 2009.

Kornfield, Jack. *The Wise Heart: A Guide to the Universal Teachings of Buddhist Psychology.* New York: Bantam Books, 2008.

Krech, Gregg. *Naikan: Gratitude, Grace, and the Japanese Art of Self-Reflection.* Berkeley: Stone Bridge Press, 2002.

Martin, Philip. *The Zen Path through Depression.* San Francisco: HarperCollins, 2000.

May, Gerald. *Addiction and Grace: Love and Spirituality in the Healing of Addictions.* New York: HarperCollins, 1988.

Merton, Thomas. *New Seeds of Contemplation.* New York: New Directions Publ., 1972.

Mother Teresa. *Come Be My Light: The Private Writings of the "Saint of Calcutta."* Ed. Brian Kolodiejchuk. New York: Doubleday, 2007.

Ortman, Dennis. *Anxiety Anonymous: The Big Book on Anxiety Addiction.* Hollister: MSI Press, 2015.

Peele, Stanton. *The Meaning of Addiction: Compulsive Experience and Its Interpretation.* Lexington: D.C. Heath and Company, 1985.

Peltz, Lawrence. *The Mindful Path to Addiction Recovery: A Practical Guide to Regaining Control over Your Life.* Boston: Shambhala, 2013.

Rohr, Richard. *Breathing Under Water: Spirituality and the Twelve Steps.* Cincinnati: St. Anthony Messenger Press, 2011.

Salzburg, Sharon. *Loving-Kindness: The Revolutionary Art of Happiness.* Boston: Shambhala, 2002.

Seligman, Martin. *Authentic Happiness.* New York: Free Press, 2002.

Shapiro, Rami. *Recovery—the Sacred Art: The Twelve Steps as Spiritual Practice.* Woodstock: SkyLight Paths Publishing, 2013.

Shenk, Joshua Wolf. *Lincoln's Melancholy: How Depression Challenged a President and Fueled His Greatness.* New York: Mariner Books, 2006.

Solomon, Andrew. *The Noonday Demon: An Atlas of Depression.* New York: Scribner, 2001.

Styron, William. *Darkness Visible: A Memoir of Madness.* New York: Vintage Books, 1990.

Tao Te Ching. Tr. Stephen Mitchell. New York: Harper Perennial Classics, 2000.

Thich Nhat Hanh. *Being Peace.* Berkeley: Parallax Press, 1987.

Twelve Steps and Twelve Traditions. New York: Alcoholics Anonymous World Services, 2012.

Williams, M., Teasdale, J., Segal, Z., and Kabat-Zin, J. *The Mindful Way through Depression: Freeing Yourself from Chronic Unhappiness.* New York: Guilford Press, 2007.

Select MSI Books

Self-Help Books

A Woman's Guide to Self-Nurturing (Romer)

Anxiety Anonymous: The Big Book on Anxiety Addiction (Ortman)

Creative Aging: A Baby Boomer's Guide to Successful Living (Vassiliadis & Romer)

Divorced! Survival Techniques for Singles over Forty (Romer)

Living Well with Chronic Illness (Charnas)

Publishing for Smarties: Finding a Publisher (Ham)

Survival of the Caregiver (Snyder)

The Marriage Whisperer: How to Improve Your Relationship Overnight (Pickett)

The Rose and the Sword: How to Balance Your Feminine and Masculine Energies (Bach & Hucknall)

The Widower's Guide to a New Life (Romer)

Widow: A Survival Guide for the First Year (Romer)

Inspirational and Religious Books

A Believer-Waiting's First Encounters with God (Mahlou)

A Guide to Bliss: Transforming Your Life through Mind Expansion (Tubali)

El Poder de lo Transpersonal (Ustman)

Everybody's Little Book of Everyday Prayers (MacGregor)

Joshuanism (Tosto)

Puertas a la Eternidad (Ustman)

The Gospel of Damascus (O. Imady)

The Seven Wisdoms of Life: A Journey into the Chakras (Tubali)

When You're Shoved from the Right, Look to Your Left: Metaphors of Islamic Humanism (O. Imady)

Memoirs

Blest Atheist (Mahlou)

Forget the Goal, the Journey Counts . . . 71 Jobs Later (Stites)

Healing from Incest: Intimate Conversations with My Therapist (Henderson & Emerton)

It Only Hurts When I Can't Run: One Girl's Story (Parker)

Las Historias de Mi Vida (Ustman)

Losing My Voice and Finding Another (C. Thompson)

Of God, Rattlesnakes, and Okra (Easterling)

Road to Damascus (E. Imady)

Still Life (Mellon)

Foreign Culture

Syrian Folktales (M. Imady)

The Rise and Fall of Muslim Civil Society (O. Imady)

The Subversive Utopia: Louis Kahn and the Question of National Jewish Style in Jerusalem (Sakr)

Thoughts without a Title (Henderson)

Popular Psychology

Road Map to Power (Husain & Husain)

The Seeker (Quinelle)

Understanding the People around You: An Introduction to Socionics (Filatova)

Humor

Mommy Poisoned Our House Guest (C. B. Leaver)

The Musings of a Carolina Yankee (Amidon)

Parenting

365 Teacher Secrets for Parents: Fun Ways to Help Your Child in Elementary School (McKinley & Trombly)

How to Be a Good Mommy When You're Sick (Graves)

Lessons of Labor (Aziz)

www.ingramcontent.com/pod-product-compliance
Lightning Source LLC
LaVergne TN
LVHW082144140625
813893LV00015B/884